This Is Me

By

Elizabeth Banes

Dedication

I would like to dedicate this book to anyone who is diagnosed with Spina Bifida or any other disability or birth defect. This is your reminder to never give up and never let anyone tell you no. You are stronger than your biggest enemy.

Acknowledgement

I first want to start off by thanking my Girl Scout mentor Pat Coyne and all of the committee volunteers for helping me get through this process and helping me reach the goal of my Gold Award. Secondly, my book editor Norma for guiding me through writing my book and helping me organize it. Also, to my family who have supported me and continue to help me throughout my whole life and through this long process, especially my parents and brother who have pushed me my whole life and taught me how to overcome many obstacles and have stood by my side no matter what we have encountered. Lastly, my friends, girl scout troop and girl scout leaders, Jen and Tammy, who have accepted me and helped me become the person I am today and who have done this crazy life with me. Every single person that I have met in my life has had a small part in my life and because of them I can be who I am.

About the Author

Born and raised in Beaver Dam. I am a 2023 Beaver Dam High school graduate, continuing my education at Bemidji State University in the Fall of 2023. I have one older brother, Noah, and two dogs: Sydney and Gino, and a cat Tiggs. I love the outdoors, hiking, swimming, running, kayaking, etc. as well as playing sports and going to sporting events. My family owns Willow Mill Campsite in Rio WI, which has been in our family for 3 generations. I am not a girly girl and I don't mind getting down and dirty and doing most things girls may not like to. I don't take no for an answer and try to prove everyone wrong everyday.

Table of Contents

Scars Tell Stories

At just twenty weeks pregnant, my parents got a triple screen test done that checked for Down Syndrome, Spina Bifida, and Edwards Syndrome. The results came back that I had Spina Bifida which prompted the doctors to have a second test done because sometimes they can come back as a false positive. When the second test came back, they knew that I did indeed have it. At that point all they wanted to know was how to help me progress forward until I was born.

My condition of Spina Bifida (called Myelomeningocele) occurs when parts of the spinal cord and nerves come through an open part of the spine causing nerve damage and fluid on the brain. Most babies have surgery at birth to stitch up the wound wherever it may be. Throughout my mom's pregnancy, the doctors monitored my back, and my body as a whole, so they were aware of what it was like. Thankfully, my wound was on the lowest part of my back which is the best position because, if it were higher up towards the neck, it would have caused paralysis. As soon as I was born, via C-section, I was taken to the NICU (Neonatal Intensive Care Unit) and the doctors said that I would have surgery later that night. So, nine hours after I was born, I had my first surgery. This surgery closed up the opening so the nerves were no longer exposed. It lasted 2 hours and went smoothly.

I was then required to have physical therapy. The therapy helped heal and strengthen my body and kept it developing and growing. However, it only lasted until I was three years old. So, when I was 3, my parents were nervous and unsure of what I would be able to do for therapy. Knowing that having exercise was beneficial to me, they continued to look for options. They soon discovered swimming lessons at Wayland Academy, a private school in Beaver Dam. Going into the first lesson, we didn't know what to expect. Would I love it or hate it? Gratefully, it was the best thing for me to continue strengthening my bones and muscles to help me grow. I had 2 lessons a week for 1 hour. We took the very first steps that would lead to years of lessons. After the first couple years learning how to swim and float in the water and have fun, I advanced to a group where I learned the breaststroke, backstroke, freestyle, butterfly, etc. and how to dive off the diving platform. Every Tuesday and Thursday after school I eagerly would go to swimming lessons and jump into that freezing cold water everyone dreaded. I loved swimming, learning new strokes, and seeing the progress from where I started to what I could do. I would say that my favorite stroke I learned was the breaststroke. It was more arm work than leg work and I just absolutely dominated it. Every now and then my grandparents, aunt and cousins, parents, and brother would come and cheer me on in races. It was a blast. Due to the lack of leg strength I had, I used my arms a lot and therefore gained a lot of arm strength. I became such a good swimmer that whenever I would swim at my parents' campground, I was called "Fishy" by some of the campers. Swimming has helped make me stronger and my love for swimming is still the same.

At six weeks old, I was diagnosed with Hydrocephalus (fluid on the brain that doesn't drain like a "normal" person's body.) So I had my second surgery. A shunt was placed in my head along with a tube that drains the fluid down to my stomach to relieve pressure off my brain and prevent life-threatening problems. Something that can come with having a shunt is a *shunt malfunction*. A shunt malfunction is when a shunt stops draining fluid and the fluid builds up and causes you to feel horrible. You can get a headache, become nauseous, fatigued and confused. Shunts are not meant to last forever and there are people who need a replacement every 3 or 4 years. So far, I have not needed a replacement but I did need a tap to "reactivate" it. When my shunt malfunctioned, I felt "under the weather," lethargic, cried constantly and had a headache for a couple days. My parents rushed me to the hospital where I had a procedure called "tapping the shunt" and immediately I felt like myself again. I perked up and was my little energetic self. Since then I have had no problems with it and have not had to replace it.

I know that I am very fortunate to have had only a few surgeries so far in my life because there are a lot of kids/adults with my disability who have 10 to 20+ surgeries. With that being said, I know that anything can happen at any time.

A Journey of a Thousand Steps Begins with a Single Step

When I turned 2 years old, Carol, my physical therapist from the Dodge County Birth to 3 program, came to my house with a walker to help me start learning to walk. Carol told my parents that it could take a while for me to get used to the walker and that it may not be easy to maneuver right away. Typical of me, I was different! I used it to pull myself up. I grabbed on to it and started moving right away. I took a loop around our couch then out in the hallway like it was nothing and went back to my parents. I sure shocked them all.

After receiving my walker, the daycare staff wanted an easier and safer way for me to get in and out of the building, so they installed a ramp at the main entrance and at the entrance to the playground to allow me to use my walker to get in and out of the building. The goal was to take my walker to daycare to help me walk and get around, but I refused to use it. The teachers decided to call my parents to ask them to pick it up because it was becoming a safety hazard for all the other kids since they wanted to use it to move around the classroom. I felt comfortable without it and didn't want it to slow me down. For some people, a phone call like that may seem mean or inconsiderate but my parents were proud that I was able to walk independently. They were so grateful that I had completed one of the uncertain milestones: Will I be able to walk? To this day I have never used a walker again, but I do use braces for balance and stability. From the beginning my parents were told that the best that I would be able to do was walk with a walker, so I know how fortunate I am to have to only wear braces. There are many kids and adults with Spina Bifida who have wheelchairs, walkers, or a combination of braces and a walker. The older I get the more I choose when I want to wear my braces. I choose to wear them for soccer and school but all my other sports and activities I choose not to wear them.

Me, Myself, and I- That's all I have at the End

Every parent enrolling their kid into school gets nervous, and sad because they don't know what to expect. Now putting a kid with a birth defect in Daycare can be even more nerve racking. It was my very first experience of being out on my own without them. Their goal for me was to always be treated like all the other kids and to be independent. They told the teachers to have "the same expectations for Elizabeth as you do any other kid." The teachers did just that. It was a great experience and a time where I was able to meet friends and focus on improving my growth. Having access to go outside gave me the opportunity to have fun and play with the kids on the playground.

I attended elementary school at South Beaver Dam. A little school in the country. At the beginning, some of the teachers and my parents had a meeting and talked about a 504 plan that they set in place for me if it were ever needed. A 504 plan is a document stating accommodations that a student may need and rules that need to be followed. I was independent and capable of doing a lot of things that I didn't ever use any of the accommodations that were listed. I always ran, played, and learned like there was nothing different because I didn't feel or notice anything different between myself and the person next to me. I played on the monkey bars and played tag. I was just a normal little kid having fun. I quickly realized that math was my favorite subject. It was the one subject where it just came easy to me. Solving equations, formulas, and problems I could always figure out. I never really had to try as hard to get a good grade. Anytime we would learn something I was able to catch on right away. During my last year I was given the opportunity to be placed in an advanced math program with my two friends, Abbey and Kendra. Once a week a teacher ran a program, and we did math that was tougher and required more thinking and problem solving.

Besides this, the only thing I did was attend a 30-minute gym session with my gym teacher to help me improve and strengthen myself. Once a week my gym teacher came in and got me from class right before our actual gym class and we worked on balance, speed, and then incorporated some fun games. Having the one on one time allowed me to learn how to adapt and adjust to get better. Every single day during gym there would be activities or games that not everyone could do or be happy about. It just shows to everyone it isn't just them, but everyone who struggles with something.

The switch from elementary school to middle school is pretty big. You are not only going to a bigger setting but also to a setting with more kids, walking and expectations. With that being said, we kept my 504 plan in place because it was a first and a concern for all of us. However as I started adapting and becoming older I soon started to realize my capabilities and still never wanted to use it. Our middle school had 3 levels and stairs to get up to the different levels. I had never experienced what it was like walking up and down that many stairs before and especially with textbooks, notebooks, etc. in my arms, so I just took it day by day.

"How would it be for me to climb the stairs with books?" "What about the other kids being on the stairs with me?" These were some thoughts that both my parents and teachers were questioning when going over the plan.

Thankfully, most of the 6th grade classes were down on the first level so I didn't have to worry about the stairs. While that wasn't a concern, gym testing was something that we knew would be a little more difficult! I knew that sit-ups would be a challenge and they were because I am unable to have movement in my toes and ankle that would've allowed me to push my feet into the ground when I curled up. On the other hand, other tests were where I was able to show my strength and abilities. The one I always looked forward to was the push up test; I usually got 25+ pushups. Funny enough, one time myself and 4 of my other friends in the class went up to the mats together and you had to follow a recording of a guy. After the guy said down, all of us went down. As he said "up", I was the only one who came up. We all started laughing, making it difficult for me to focus on the recording. However, I composed myself and kept going. Any other day of class, I participated and tried my hardest whether it was volleyball, roller skating, rock climbing, scooters, etc. I had a fun time and never slowed down.

Our 7th grade classes were on the very top floor of the three-story school, with the gym and music rooms on the first floor. In order to get from gym to class and class to gym, I had to take the stairs. Within my 504 plan it stated that I was allowed to use the elevator to make it to class on time and prevent me from potentially getting bumped by other kids on the stairs. I liked walking up and down the stairs because it made me feel the same. I felt that if I took the elevator kids would see me differently and I would feel guilty because I am more than capable of taking the stairs. There were plenty of other kids that took the elevator for fun or to be lazy but it never even came to my mind all three years of being in middle school. To me it is seen as something that someone needs if they physically cannot get up the stairs (like in a wheelchair or on crutches, etc.). Whereas I was physically capable of walking up the stairs with my books in my hands. I was able to enjoy the time with my friends and others by taking time to walk the stairs with them. My most enjoyable times in my first two years of middle school were always my math classes because I loved the two teachers I had and how they engaged us all in group activities with our table mates to solve equations.

By the time I got to 8th grade I realized how far I was able to walk, the more I was able to push myself in testing and school work in general and knew that I didn't need anything to help me be successful. I needed myself and my confidence. By being independent and learning to not use the elevator to get around I was able to prepare for high school. It showed me what I needed to expect because once high school started I knew that there was going to be a lot of walking to different classes.

Once high school started for me many big milestones occurred that changed me into a better, more educated and well-rounded individual. Starting out, my goal was to figure out the layout of the school, where all my classes were to manage my time to make sure I made it to class on time and to get comfortable with the amount of classwork and homework I would receive. It was recently remodeled to one level when I had gotten there so it made it easier to navigate. There was no talk about getting rid of my 504 plan and with being new to the school we still kept it just like all the other years, even though we knew that it was never really used. It just helped inform the teachers of what they could do in class and what they weren't allowed to have in class, i.e. balloons or anything latex. Interestingly enough, all 4 years of high school, my locker has been located in the far end of the school, away from the main door, so every day I have a long walk. Intentionally, I would say it has been close to most of my classes which makes it more convenient and gives me the ability to take multiple notebooks/textbooks with me and stopping at my locker either 1 or 2 times a day. I wasn't really nervous going to high school for the walking, more so the size and course work I would have to do. I signed up to take my first honors class ever; Honors Geometry. I had taken Algebra 1 in 8th grade so I was already past that first class that most kids would take freshman year so I had a choice. I could either take geometry or Honors Geometry and the teacher recommended Honors Geometry, which I chose. I didn't know what to expect but my grades in math before were excellent. Well, Honors Geometry was a huge speed bump in my liking for math and it coming to me easily.

They say that you either understand algebra or geometry more. I quickly realized algebra was more my type because that geometry class really hit me hard. I'll admit I struggled. I wasn't doing as well as I had done my whole life. I was struggling to learn the material in class and apply it to my homework which then made the tests that much more difficult. I was able to complete my homework with the help of friends, my knowledge and the teacher. Getting credit for my homework helped so when I didn't do well on the tests, which was mostly all of them, I was able to still have a decent grade in the class. However, I had gone into the class hoping for better. My least favorite thing I learned how to do was proofs. If you couldn't get one step, all of the other steps to solve it right were also most likely going to be wrong. I rarely was able to figure out how to get all of the right steps in the right order.

A Difficult class + not being able to do so well + new to high school = my love for math slowly diminished.

I started not looking forward to the class, not wanting to go because I knew I wasn't going to do well in it. I persevered, went in during WIN time to get assistance and ended with a high B-. Not terrible, but also not my greatest either.

When the next school year approached I had Honors Algebra 2 as my next math class to take. Since I struggled in geometry, I was not really excited or sure what the class would be like. After a couple days in it though I realized it was true; Honors Algebra 2 was easier again for me. My brain was able to click right away. I understood the lessons we were doing. The equations were just like what Algebra 1 had, just more steps or more in depth. My love for math was coming back and I was excited for math class every day. I had an amazing teacher that

I loved, Mr. Chase. He made learning fun and always allowed us to work with others. My grade showed that I understood the content and it was amazing. There was one hard lesson within Algebra 2 that I will absolutely never love and that is trigonometry. It was my only bad test score in that class for the entire year.

We all go through growth and change especially during our sophomore to junior years.

That is exactly what happened to me. A lot was starting to unfold near the end of my sophomore year. I turned 15 ½ and was eligible to get my driving temps. I would soon have the freedom to drive wherever I wanted without my parents in the car with me, but first I had to watch videos and take a test to pass.

Growing up I never thought of having a difficult time driving given my ankle movement limitations but it was brought up a couple times at my doctor visits that I go to yearly. I can assure you that having Spina Bifida or anything doesn't have to stop you from being able to have the experience of driving but you may just have to adjust to what your capabilities are. However not everyone with a birth defect or circumstance is lucky enough to have the opportunity to drive like me. My type of Spina Bifida prevents me from being able to have the ability to move my ankle and feet including my toes making it difficult to press the brake/gas down with the feeling of complete control. They mentioned that it would be a good idea to get into a special driving school that gave me extra assistance with driving to make it easier for me and there were options where I could get special pedals and different equipment, but I knew that I would be able to adjust slightly and not need any equipment.

All of my videos I watched were online and I took the end of video quizzes from my phone. Unpopular opinion, but I found those videos interesting and would sit in my room and do 2 or 3 videos and quizzes a night. Once my video lessons were completed I scheduled an in person time to go take the official quiz to get my temps and start behind the wheel to get my actual licenses. Days leading up to the quiz I was taking practice quizzes that were provided and was getting pretty confident with the knowledge. I took it and passed and I was onto the behind the wheel. My behind-the-wheel experience was not traditional because Covid was present and we were unable to have people closely together in a car. So I was the only one in the car with the instructor and we had to have our temperature taken before we got in the car and we had to put on hand sanitizer, gloves and wear a mask. The lessons lasted an hour only and I didn't have to observe anyone else. They consisted of the basic maneuvers and looks, parallel parking, y turn, 3 point turn, parking in stalls, etc. I loved my instructor, Cindy, she was amazing. Then one day we went out for a lesson and she told me where to go and we pulled up to a storage unit and I had no idea what was happening. She told me she only did this for the kids she felt were ready and super good drivers; I had to back up around a storage unit. It truly wasn't as bad it may seem at first. From the beginning we knew that my case of Spina Bifida was the best case scenario and it continued to be shown while driving. To start out I would check my speed on the speedometer every few minutes but over time I have gotten used to it and it has become more natural. I am capable of pushing on the brakes without slamming them down. I stay as controlled and smooth behind the wheel as much as possible and keep aware of my surroundings so that if I have passengers they feel safe and know that I am a responsible and capable driver. Spina Bifida doesn't prevent me from getting the opportunities that everyone else is given in their lives. I don't see my disability as something to be ashamed of or a negative aspect of my life. It has taught me how to be creative, think outside the box and do anything that anyone else is doing.

When I thought my sophomore year couldn't get any better it did. I started to get the hang of school and my grades were reflecting it. I always strived to have the best grades possible and near the end of that year I was inducted into our school's National Honor Society. Most schools have a National Honor Society but not all of them have the same requirements to get in. Our school's requirement is that you have to have a 3.5 GPA or higher to qualify to be eligible to be inducted starting your sophomore year of high school. When I was a sophomore, I received a letter saying that I qualified to be eligible for the National Honor Society. I had the right GPA and was a perfect candidate. The letter explained why I was eligible. There were application papers included. The applications are read by a committee and they choose who is inducted into the NHS. The application required information that included: service activities, employment, and clubs and organizations (both in and out of school.) I also had to write an essay explaining an event in my life that I have had to overcome, or that changed me, and how I show proper PRIDE at our school. At the deadline of when the application was due, our advisor took them to the next step. A group of teachers went through the stack and reviewed the applications. About 25 people of the 50 were chosen. Two weeks later, we were supposed to receive an email if we were inducted. Relieved, I received the email at school but waited until I had gotten home to open the email. It was worth the wait because after I got home, the email read, "Congratulations you have been selected for the National Honor Society." Happy as ever, I couldn't wait until the weekend to tell the rest of my family. Finally, the weekend came and I was able to tell my grandma and grandpa that I got in. "Wow, that's awesome!" they said. "Congratulations! That's huge. None of us have been in it." The email also said the date of the induction ceremony.

The day of the ceremony came and we were told to dress nice and no jeans or shorts. At the ceremony, the names were listed in alphabetical order so my name was the second one called on the list. I walked in front of the stage, up the steps, then walked across the stage to our advisor at the time, Mr. Pogorelic. He shook my hand, handed me my certificate and pin, and said, "Congratulations." I sat down in the next empty chair on the stage and the other names were called. Roughly 20 kids later, we were all told to stand and say the NHS pledge, which we promised to give our best and to do our service duties. After the pledge we exited the stage, row after row, and went into the cafeteria where our families waited to celebrate. When I got by my family they all congratulated me and started taking photos with me, and my certificate. What made the ceremony extra special is that I was also able to celebrate it with two of my best friends that I have had since kindergarten and before: Kendra and Abbey.

Excited to start NHS but unaware of what it entirely entailed, I went to my "first" meeting of the year. At the first meeting I learned the amount of service hours needed and that every month, our group would meet to discuss service projects we were going to host and do as a NHS group. Other meetings were just check-ins and discussions talking about what it means to represent Beaver Dam High School. To continue to be a part of the NHS, there are certain rules that you have to follow otherwise you can be removed from it. The first one includes maintaining the 3.5 GPA or higher. Second, you have to attend the meetings when they are scheduled, and you are only allowed to have three unexcused absences. The first unexcused is a warning, the second is 2 extra service hours and the third is a talk with the advisor and the reviewers where they will discuss and see if they want you removed or not. My very first meeting experience was not the best and one I still regret to this day. I made a mistake. I hadn't joined the google classroom that the advisor had sent us that had the schedule of when the meetings were. I was then unable to see the messages and didn't get the message that there was a meeting that morning. I went to school and my friend asked me where I was. "What do you mean?" I asked her. "There was an NHS meeting this morning," she replied. As soon as she told me that there had been a meeting and I missed it, it never left my mind. I immediately emailed my advisor and apologized because I felt so bad. She replied with "This is a warning."

Throughout the whole day I was upset thinking about missing the meeting. I thought I was going to cry. I knew the only thing that I could do was to not miss another meeting. I accepted my mistake and moved on, making all the meetings the rest of the year.

"When you make a mistake, there are only three things you should ever do about it: admit it, learn from it, and don't repeat it."

- Paul Bear Bryant

The Veterans Day ceremony we hold every year is my favorite thing about being in the National Honor Society. It is the very first service event that we hold every year and it is for the Veterans in the community. We decorate the auditorium with streamers, banners, and balloons and the cafeteria area with patriotic stars, table cloths, and table toppers to showcase our love for their sacrifice. The most recent ceremony that we held, the veterans were able to come early in the morning and then, as members, we talked and interacted with them until breakfast was served. Talking with the veterans and hearing all the different branches that these men and women were a part of was interesting. There was such a variety of stories. I remember specifically one guy told me that our generation coming up is the reason why those men and women did what they did. He said that they don't do it for themselves, they do it for the generations that follow. Many stories later, the veterans headed to the auditorium where the ceremony took place. After the ceremony, the veterans left and we got back to class after getting everything cleaned up. The ceremonies are so special and enjoyable. I am happy to be able to interact with them all and hear about how they risked their lives for us to be happy and free.

Change, change, and more change. Junior year when I took Applied Graphics I was starting to think that I was in love with designing and creating cool things. It was the third level of the design class and my skills were improving. I was becoming more creative and came out with really cool projects that I was able to create myself. There were three of us in the class and we worked together a lot to make items for our school store, such as graduation year keychains, t-shirts, sweatshirts, cups, etc. We were able to also make things for us to have as a memory for the class.

My favorite project that we did was a laser burn on a wooden slab. I didn't really know if I wanted to make it for myself, something with adventure or sports or my pets, or if I wanted to surprise my parents and make it for the campground. After a lot of brainstorming and researching, I decided to make one for myself and one for my parents. I was proud of the sign I made for the campground. I had the idea to recreate the lake with some chairs and a fire, then incorporate the signature willow tree in it as well. To make it even more original, I added the name of the campground, the year it was established and then added a unique border. I was so proud of how that came out and I decided to create one for myself as well. I made it represent me, with a cliff, water and a quote that says "Don't predict the future, create it." Both designs came out just like I had wanted and when I showed my parents their slab they were in love.

They displayed it at the campground and so many people had complimented it and asked if I was selling it or could make some. Hearing that makes me love that I did the project even more. Also that year I took strength and conditioning, as my gym class, to become more ready for my powerlifting and soccer season. I didn't modify or change anything to help me succeed differently in the class or to make anything easier, besides if we were doing band work due to my latex allergy. I ran the intervals, including 20, 100 meter intervals every other day, lifted weights, did pull ups, 30 meter dash, etc. There were some exercises that were more challenging because of my lack of balance control but I never used it as an excuse to not try.

There were plenty of kids who just did the class to get an "easy" grade or to hang out with their friends, but I was there to get stronger and more fit for sports. I adjusted, kept trying, and improved by the end of the semester-long class. Every lift was not mega amounts of weight but as I grew I was working on my techniques and focusing on me and my capability. It was me vs. me and nobody else. The teachers recognized how much I was improving and so was I. I was happy with my growth from the start to the end.

On the flip side, there's always something about school that makes a lot of kids not want to go and that is classes they are not very fond of participating in. My least favorite class is History/Government, etc. I have never been the one to really like learning about what happened way, way before I was born. I am not disagreeing that it is important to learn what happened to the people and places before I existed but it doesn't interest me. I would rather just focus on what happened in the recent past and how it is effecting what is going on now. With that being said, it is also just physically harder for me to retain information like that and the years that things happened and who was involved in actions or discoveries. There are definitely things that do intrigue me about history but I would rather just learn about current events. An event that I like hearing about that occurred in the past is 9-11. It was obviously a horrible event that happened that everybody remembers and something we hope never happens again. For me it is easy to comprehend and therefore something interesting for me to learn about. Every year we do a remembrance lesson and go over what happened, how everybody responded and what it's like now.

In a blink of an eye from being a little baby not knowing how my life ahead was going to look to now, being a senior in high school, a part of so many activities, sports, and clubs.

Looking back there is nothing that I regret doing and everything I did then has prepared me for the future that is fast approaching. As I am finishing up high school and have turned into an adult I have had the responsibility of looking at future plans both academically and life-wise.

College has always been something that I knew that I wanted to pursue after high school but up until searching schools I didn't know what I would go for. While searching for colleges I came across the major Kinesiology/Exercise Science and immediately after reading what it was I knew that that was exactly what I wanted to do. I continued my search for colleges that were good for Kinesiology in and near Wisconsin and I found some colleges that I was interested in touring. I narrowed my options to four schools that I wanted to tour and this past summer we made it a priority to take a trip to look at them. The very first college that we toured was University of Wisconsin- Madison. I was so excited to tour this college, for many different reasons. I have grown up going to both badger hockey games and badger volleyball games. I love the culture/atmosphere that you feel and experience while watching them. Everyone is always rooting and supporting the teams and I just enjoy going every time. By touring the campus this summer it felt like a side of Madison that I hadn't experienced yet, and I loved it. I knew that if I put it all together it was going to be something that I would enjoy. On the tour they gave us an inspirational speech and then took us around part of the campus and showed us some of the buildings and discussed classes you would take there. The best and my most favorite part of the tour was going down by the lake, to the Memorial Union and hearing how kids go down there all the time and study for exams or do their homework. It truly felt like home to me. I left there satisfied with my first college tour experience. My next college that I visited was University of Wisconsin- Eau Claire. It's a little bit further away from home but the campus was smaller and enclosed. It was also beautiful. We had another informational meeting at the beginning and then were sent out with a current student who gave us a tour. We were able to actually go inside the buildings and see what a classroom would look like and a lecture hall. It made it feel more realistic and I was able to see what I would be like in one of those classrooms. Another difference between the tours from Madison to Eau Claire was that we were able to see a dorm room that incoming college freshmen and sophomores would have to live in while on campus. They were small, but normal dorm rooms.

After touring those two colleges, Madison was still my favorite and constantly always on my mind of where I was going to go. However, I wanted to tour more and have more contenders to pair with Madison so my final two choices were University of Wisconsin- La Crosse and Bemidji State University. If I am being completely honest, I wasn't too excited to go to La Crosse and Eau Claire but I still went. When we went to La Crosse there were quite a lot of kids who were also wanting the tour. We got the same presentation as the other ones of their acceptance rate, what it required to get in, majors/minors, etc. It was shocking to me how much I was enjoying it. Then we got on the tour of the campus. The size of the campus I would say is medium to small and not that spread out. All the classes were in the same area with decent amounts of walking. We were able to go inside the classrooms and see lecture halls and experience the dorm rooms that they had there. Leaving there, La Crosse was definitely on my possible list of colleges. Last but not least, my mom and I drove 7.5 hours to Bemidji, Minnesota to tour Bemidji State University. This was the tour that I was most excited for, besides Madison. We drove up two days before the tour so that the day before we would be able to explore the area a little bit and get a feel for what it could look like to be there. We had a hotel right on the lake and it was amazing. We went on a walk and just took in the beauty. We went and drove past the university and instantly I saw that it was a great combination between Madison and La Crosse. The surrounding area had the feel of Madison, busy, food places, a mall/shops, but the campus itself was off of the main road and medium to small sized with amazing views of Bemidji Lake. That night, after driving around and seeing the sights, I knew that there may have been a reason that I was drawn to Bemidji. We found a BBQ place and then walked to get some ice cream. Once back at the hotel we went in the pool and then headed off to bed. The next morning was the morning of the tour. We got up early to go for a walk/run on the trail before we got ready to head over. When we arrived at the university we went into the ballroom and sat at a table and waited for the presentation to start. The presentation was so engaging and interactive that it made it fun. We were able to respond to the questions they had on the board on our phones and see everyone's responses pop up on the screen. This school's campus tour was my favorite out of all the tours. We were able to go into some of the school buildings and classrooms and see the dorm rooms. The views from each classroom and walking from building to building were just amazing, with the water and the scenery around the campus. We were also very lucky to see their recreational building where the track, basketball courts, indoor tennis court and workout equipment was. It was all so cool. The information that they provided us with was worth everything. I left that day happy and having a big decision to make on where I want to pursue my college education. After thinking about all of the tours I had attended I decided that I would eliminate Eau Claire from my list, so I just focused on applying to Bemidji, Madison and La Crosse. The very first school I got accepted to was Bemidji and the moment I found out that I was accepted I was excited, it felt like a surreal moment. The next acceptance I got was to La Crosse. Currently, I am waiting for Madison. I have been thinking about my options and trying to pick the best school that will benefit me in the long run. Each of the schools have their pros and cons but I know deep down I will be happy with whatever choice I make. Being able to go and experience these college tours with my parents was fun and a great experience that I really enjoyed doing. Now, the next thing I need to do is continue my path to the career of my dreams and see where my life goes after high school.

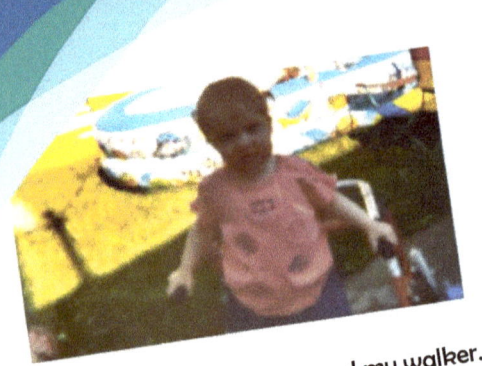

One of the very few times I used my walker.

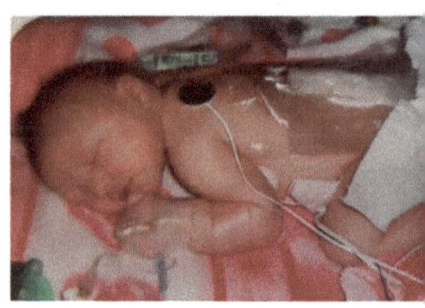

The day I was born, right after my surgery.

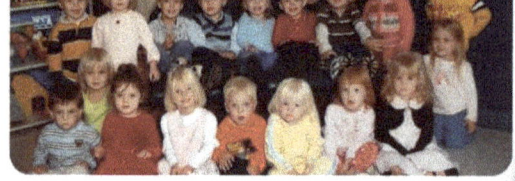

My Daycare schoolmates

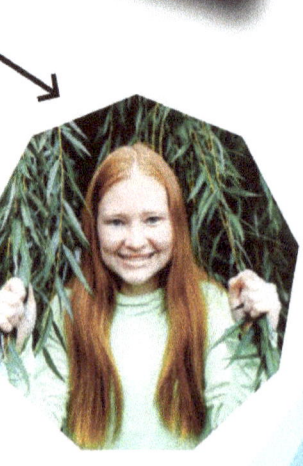

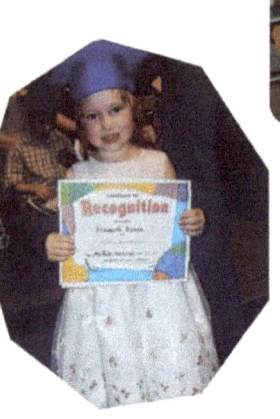

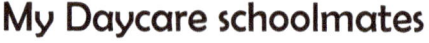

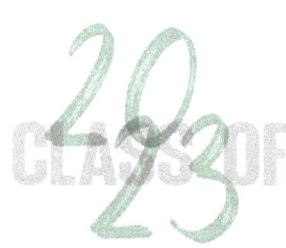

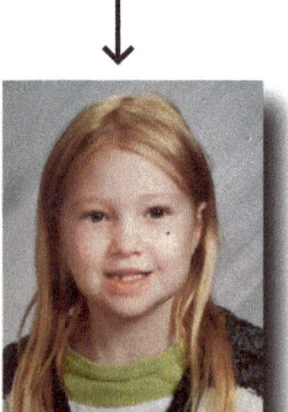

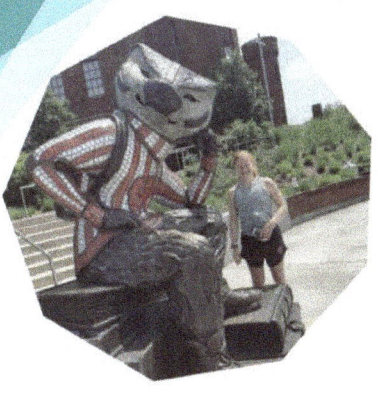

Standing next to a bucky badger statue on my tour to UW-Madison.

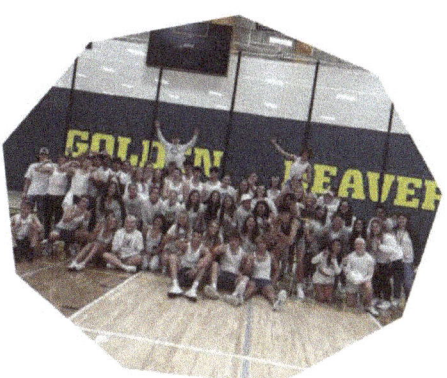

Senior classmates after a Macho Man victory during Homecoming.

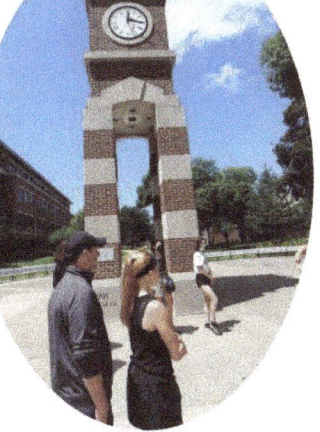

Clock tower on my tour to UW- Lacrosse.

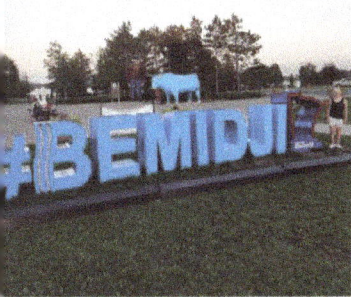

#Bemidji sign on my tour to Bemidji State University ith Paul and Babe in the back.

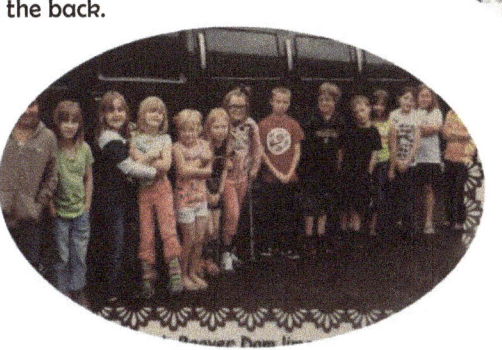

Limbo at recess in Elementary school.

Line of kids who rode in the Limo at school for selling a certain amount of items for a fundraiser.

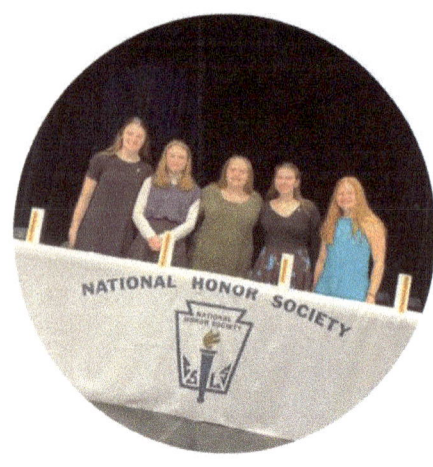

Abbey, McKenzie, Jordyn, Kendra, and I after Jordyn's induction night.

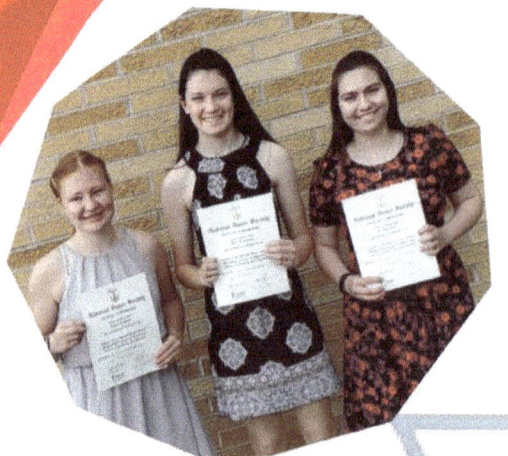

Me, Abbey, and Kendra after National Honor Society induction night.

NATIONAL HONOR SOCIETY

National Honor Society
Certificate of Membership
This certifies that
Elizabeth Banes
was selected as a member of the

Chapter of the National Honor Society.
Membership is based on Scholarship,
Service, Leadership, and Character.

Presented at Beaver Dam High School

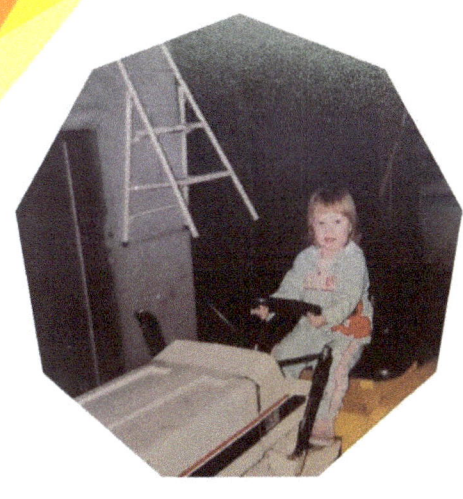

Riding Mower Driver

Boat Driver

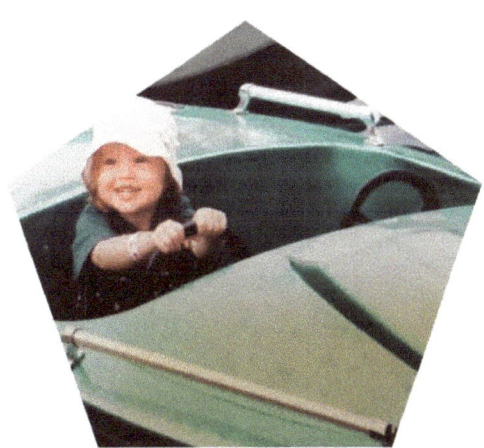

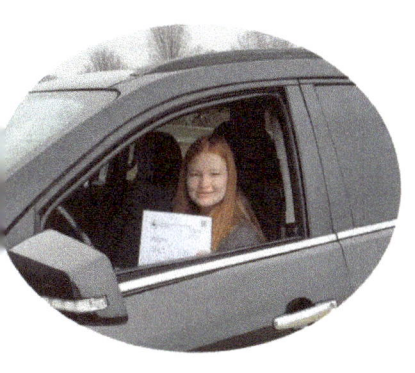

As soon as I got home
after getting my temps.

My 16th birthday with
my printed license.

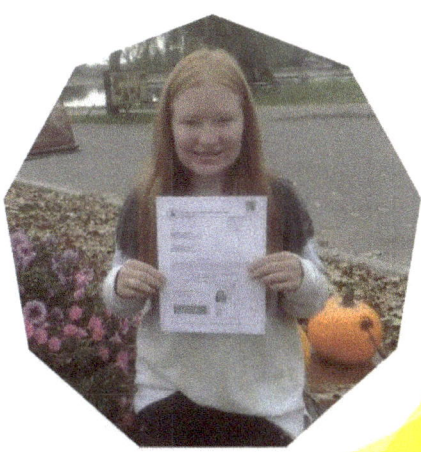

Grit for Gold

Sports have always been a part of my family. My dad grew up playing hockey, my mom played softball and basketball when she was younger and my brother was also in sports at a very young age, so I grew up around the sports culture. At the age of 4 my parents had signed me up for T-ball through the Beaver Dam Parks, Rec and Forestry. It was a great way to not only meet kids and make friends but it was also great exercise for me. I enjoyed it and my parents had fun watching me. That was officially my first sport.

My very first sport that I actually have memories of participating in is soccer. A couple years prior to my 5th grade year I had talked a little bit about wanting to play soccer, but nothing was ever a 100% type of thing. Then one night in 5th grade I told my parents "I want to join soccer." They responded with "ok, we will look at getting you signed up for the club team." So, they signed me up and I joined. You may think that since my brother was playing and I was always at every game that I would know all of the terminology but I didn't. I had gone to my first practice knowing basic things like positions and how to play but I didn't understand offsides, advantages, etc. When we arrived my dad talked to my coaches and mentioned my birth defect and that I had to wear braces and all they just said was "ok, we'll adjust if we need to." They understood. Throughout that first practice I started learning more and more about the game and getting comfortable with my teammates and playing with my braces and learning how to kick the ball and run with it. The rest of the season was super fun and I learned a lot and grew as an individual and a player. We didn't win any games, but I learned the concept of the game and how to work with a team of players. I also figured out the position that was my favorite and I played throughout my whole school playing career; DEFENSE. During middle school I continued to play soccer but these years were different. We had new coaches and a few new players. Most of the players had just moved up the next age level like I did but not all.

Within the 3 years a lot changed both physically and mentally for me. From the beginning we were winning more games, the coaches were teaching us how and when to move on the field depending on where the ball was, we were told to communicate and talk as a group and I was evolving as an individual to make my team better. The coaches had practiced a lot with us and were giving us pointers and strategies during practice that we implemented into the games. We connected as a team better than any of my other years playing. I even experienced my first ball to the face. The only thing I remember is standing still in the back on the line of defense and then all of a sudden the ball came straight for the left side of my face. Instead of going down and being hurt, I shook it off and ran to defend the ball from the other team. The game continued and I played on. Once the game finished everyone made sure I was ok including my mom and my friend's mom, Tammy. They told me how much of a warrior I am for continuing to play like nothing happened.

My most fond memories from middle school soccer were tournaments. One of the tournaments we had played in was right after Halloween. It was called the Pumpkin tournament and we were the team that dominated the whole thing. The points were based off of goals conceded and then you got an automatic 6 points if you had scored at least 3 goals against the other team and let in 0, so every game our focus was trying to do our best and score as much as possible. We had played so well we had only conceded one goal throughout the whole thing and had scored at least 3 every game. We won 1st place. They had a trophy ceremony where we received our own individual trophies. As a defender on the team it was a pretty cool experience, being one of the players that contributed to not letting very many goals in the net was something that I know I may not have seen coming when I was just a little kid. It was the first time I had gotten a trophy! I felt so proud and accomplished.

Another tournament that I remember was with the same team a year or two later and it was one that our coaches told us in practice a couple days before was going to be hard and that winning first or even coming close to 1st place was not really promising because the competition level there of the teams was super high. As a team we didn't let that stop us. Our coaches still came out and told us what we needed to do in each game to play to our highest potential. The first day, we played multiple games: back to back and breaks between. When we had a break we rested and watched the other teams compete. It was super warm that day and while watching the other games we tried to cool ourselves off and stay hydrated for our remaining games we had left. We hadn't done as well in that tournament as our last but we did really relatively well. I don't remember exactly if we won every game leading up to our last game but we were playing for first place again in this tournament. Our competition was a good one (the number one team) and we knew they were going to be tough but we were ready and in it to win it. As one of the defenders of the team I knew that my job was to help this team win the trophy and so that game, that was my only focus. When the whistle blew and we started playing we were evenly matched. Both teams were able to keep it near the center of the field away from both goals. Fortunately, we were able to find the back of the net really early on in the game and so we were up, but a little while later they had scored to tie it up. The game continued to be a battle and we all continued to fight. We were evenly matched for each other, both teams were giving their all until the very end and the game ended in a tie so, per the rules of a tournament, we had to go into a penalty kick shootout to determine the winner.

In a penalty kick shootout every player that is on the field at the end of the game has to stay on the field. Then the players on the field are the first ones to take the penalty kicks.

However, it is usually best of 5 so you only have 5 take the pk's first. Since 11 are on the field the coaches have to choose their top 5 players.

Our coaches picked the first 5 and then the rest of us stayed off to the side on the field, cheering on our teammates. A few of our girls had gone up to the line and missed but the other team also missed some of their opportunities as well. Then it came down to the last two players; either we would make it, keep it going and the rest of us on the field would be up to take the pk or the other team would win. Our player went up to the pk spot, shot it and the ball was blocked by the goalie. All of us in disbelief and sadness walked over to the rest of the team on the bench. We lost the game, the girls who had missed their shots were the most disappointed but our coaches had gathered us in a circle and gave us a talk. They told us how well we did in the tournament and that winning second place was just as exciting and worth celebrating, they told us that we had taken this team all the way to the end and never gave up. They then awarded us with our medals and we as a team walked over to the pavilion where they awarded us our trophies. Our award ceremony was more bitter than what we wanted but looking back I am just grateful to have gotten a trophy representing what our best was at that time. Teary eyed, we all stood in a line and the head of the tournament called our names off as we received them. After all our names were called we went over as a team and got our pictures taken with our trophies and medals around our neck. No matter how hard it was to receive 2nd place over 1st, being able to come out of a tournament that we didn't think we would place in is something that I think about every time I see it because I know exactly how hard we worked that day.

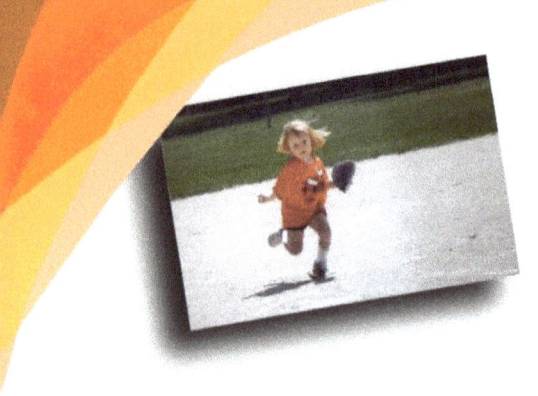

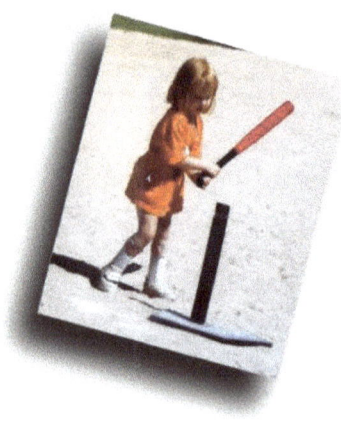

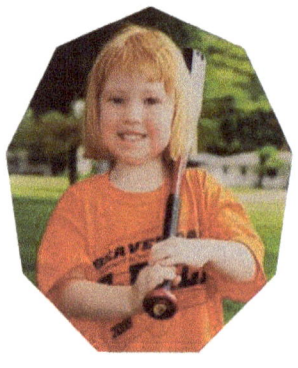

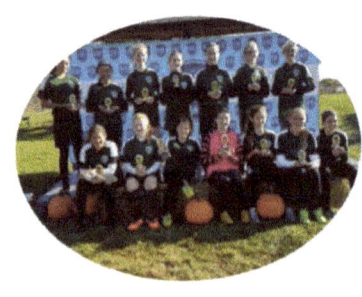

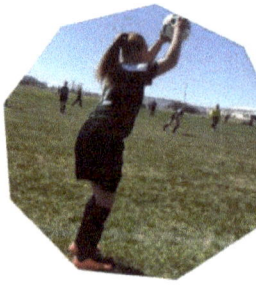

Middle School

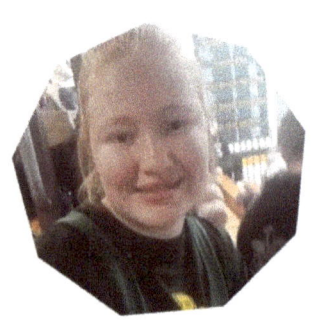

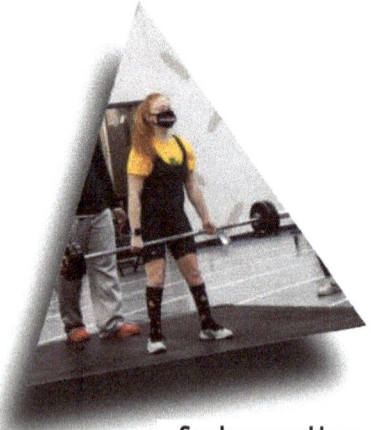

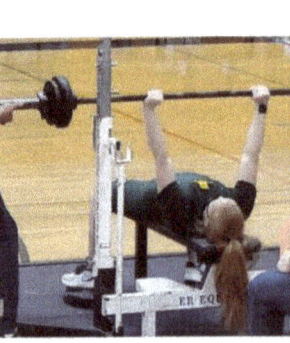

Freshman Year

Sophomore Year

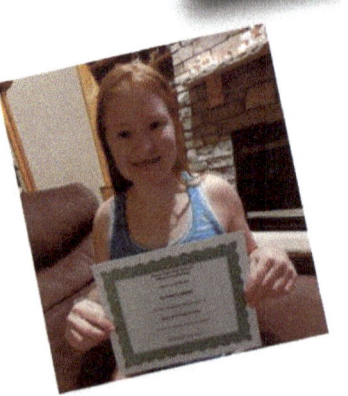

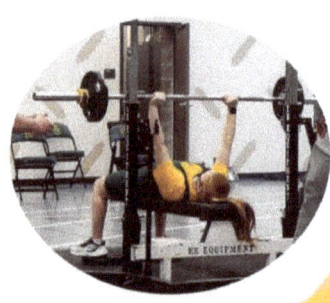

Transitioning into high school you are given so many more different clubs and sport options to do. I knew that I was going to continue soccer without a question, but I saw powerlifting and it caught my eye. I was starting to get into lifting and working out and I knew I had a great upper body. That night I told my parents that I wanted to join Powerlifting and that was the beginning of the best decision ever. A couple of weeks later, we met with the coach and got the details. I fell in love and knew that it would be good for me. However, I didn't like it when he told me that the buses left at 6 am and didn't get back until 5 pm. That winter season of my freshman year it started and I was doing it with my neighbor and friend, Nathan. I didn't know what to expect but I was excited to start it and see how far my body could go.

I quickly realized it is an all-day meet where there are about 7 different schools competing against each other. There are 4 different platforms and depending on how many kids there are usually 5 different flights (A-E). When teams first arrive, you have to go to a platform and they will have volunteers there to help you get your rack height for your squats. Once you get your rack height everyone goes to either the girls or boy's locker room and does their weigh in. After weighing in everyone goes to their designated spots and usually eats food and then if you are in the first flight, you warm up and get ready for the first event which is squat. Then they hold a lifters meeting and go over what a "clean" lift looks like and then the national anthem is played and the first flight begins. There are 3 events: **squat, bench, deadlift** and you have 3 attempts at each event. Each attempt you are allowed to go up in weight but not down. Each attempt takes about 15 seconds and your whole event takes about 5 minutes and then you are waiting for like an hour and a half to warm up for the next event. While waiting for your turn you just watch all the other competitors and eat food to fuel your body. It can be boring to wait there but it is also cool at the same time to see everyone get into it and compete.

The first meet was a nightmare. The order who goes first in the flight depends on the weight on the bar and since I was starting out with just squatting the bar it meant that I had to go first. My teammate Lily and I were sitting down in the chairs and the coach came up to us and said "Elizabeth you're first." "What, I don't know what I am doing" I say, panicking even more. He reassured me that it would be fine and that I would be able to do it, and I just had to keep my balance; which is easier said than done for me. On my first ever squat I went up to the bar and I squatted down and tried to come back up and on the way back up I lost my balance and it was a "bad" lift. Same for my second and third lift. When I got to the bench I was able to do better and get all white lights meaning I got a clean lift. A couple hours later I attempted the deadlift.

Another obstacle I had to try to get over. Unsuccessful this time I knew I would eventually get it if I kept working towards it. My very first year was hard for me because my balance wasn't the best, but I continued to show up to practice trying to figure out different strategies to help get my squats. My coach and I tried several different squat techniques but none of them seemed to work. Every competition I tried my hardest and at my very last meet of my first year I finally got my very first deadlifts. I was willing to do whatever it took to get a good squat and a good deadlift and it paid off. I was ecstatic.

The most important thing I learned was that I loved it. It was my element in being able to do something that was enjoyable and fun but that challenged me. I felt like it was benefiting my body in a good way and I liked how it made me feel. I felt potential if I came back the next season. However soon after that Covid hit and shut us all down. I was so excited to start soccer but unfortunately at the time it got delayed and so instead of it affecting me and making me lazy, I decided to invest in my health with hopes we would have a soccer season, which we obviously didn't, and start running. Being in quarantine allowed me to have time for running during the day. My daily routine consisted of schoolwork in the morning and then by 11 or 12, when my mom would go out for her walk, I would go out for my run. Once I got back from the run, I would eat lunch and finish up schoolwork. I started out easy and only ran for a small distance and then progressively went farther. I was becoming happier, and healthier. I noticed changes within my body and the way I saw my life. I was happy both physically and mentally so I continued it into the summer where I kept improving and kept getting stronger and stronger. Most days it would be 90 degree weather and after work I would run around the campground. Some days I would run 2 miles or more and some days if it got too hot, I would only run for 1.5 miles. I showed up day after day no matter the weather or circumstance. If I was tired from a long day of work I would still be out crushing my goals of becoming better. It got to the point where the campers would tell me that I was insane for running in the heat but they were always proud of me. I didn't do it for them or anyone else, the only person I did it for was myself but having the encouragement and praise from them brought the fight to continue. When they thought I was crazy I would just tell them it makes me feel good, and I always had a reward for myself when I got done: swimming in the pool. When I felt more comfortable, I decided that I wanted to try to run even further distances than the 2 to 3 miles I already was repetitively doing, so I decided to train for the distance of 10k. When I would get asked if I was training for a race, I would reply, "No, just training to be able to do one on my own." Running has given me so much in my life. It changed who I am and enabled me to accomplish things that people thought weren't possible when I was born with my birth defect.

When fall/winter time came I had started training for a half marathon. I didn't want to run a half marathon but it was great for increasing my endurance. Our school had gone to a hybrid schedule; 2 days at school, 3 days virtually so I ran when I could and still was as happy as I had been during the summer. I hadn't been comparing myself to anyone or anything. During the summer, I told my parents that I wanted to do tennis and since it was fall time they signed me up and I was able to join the team a little into the season of my junior year. I had started to think of tennis as something that seemed cool and interesting for a couple years and so I thought it was going to be good to invest in. Also, having the upper body strength that I do, tennis seemed like a good thing for me. The coaches and players were very inviting and kind when I first got there. My teammates were patient and helpful in helping me learn the game and how to properly do things. I had learned a lot that year from both players and the coaches. My very first match that I played was at home and I remember I had no idea what I was doing. I had no knowledge of how to keep score, what the scoring was and any terms that were associated with tennis, not to mention the biggest thing: HOW TO SERVE. Thankfully and rightfully, I was paired up with one of my classmates Sophia who knew what she was doing. She was so patient and helpful for my first match. It made it very fun even though we lost. At the end of the first match the coach came out to the court and asked if we wanted to play another match with two more girls from the other team and we said yes and so we got to play another match and we won it. My first tennis match experience was a fun one. The rest of the year I continued to learn skills at practice and get better and improve. Fortunately, another one of my teammates, Cameran, volunteered to teach me how to serve.

Later in the year we went as a team to play Waunakee and they had all single players because of covid precautions and so we all had to play singles. I was terrified because I had never played singles before let alone just learning how to play doubles and so the coaches before I went out there just told me to have fun and try my best and that was what I did. I lost but I learned how to play something that I never knew how. I grew as an individual player which helped me be more successful in doubles. From that game on no matter who my partner was I continued to win more and more games and improve and have fun. At the end of the year, we were unable to have an award ceremony but I was awarded with my athletic participation award and very fortunate to receive the Most Improved Player award. That same summer that I decided to do tennis I was also deciding if I wanted to continue Powerlifting. I was on the fence because my friend Nathan hadn't really been into it anymore with Covid happening and so I wasn't very excited that I would be on my own but I decided to give it a try and keep going. Let me tell you, it was the best decision I made because I was able to incorporate both weight training and running into my days and I noticed a lot of changes in my body. I gained a lot of muscle in my legs and more than I had realized and mentally I was feeling better.

The meets had shrunk in time, we had to wear masks and there was our team and another team to prevent large crowds so we were able to start at 8 and we would be done by 11 in the morning. The very first meet in Laconia I reached my goal as a sophomore: **completing a good squat where I was parallel and not losing my balance on the way up or down!** We had a former girl coach from Beaver Dam warm up with us and she had given me the tip to stagger my feet so that one of them was already a tad back when I came up so if I were to lose my balance my foot was already going to be there to "catch" me. So I tried that and with focus, I was able to stick my first squat in practice! I was so excited. After warming up, we headed out to the platform and Alison spotted me from the back and I attempted just the bar and got it. My next lift I attempted 65 lbs and fell forward but I knew I could get it on my third lift and I did. Between running and strengthening my calves, quads, and staggering my feet, I believe that those things helped me get that squat I had been longing for. My deadlifts were also able to improve, and I ended up lifting 115 lbs. by the end. Similarly, my bench was still really good and I accomplished 110 lbs. The minute I got my squats and deadlifts I told my coach and he made the joke to me "What are your parents feeding you?" "Pasta," I replied excited and laughingly. It changed who I was and enabled me to accomplish things that I thought weren't possible because of the lack of balance I have compared to everyone else. It helped bring more confidence for the years after and it made me want to return to the sport for my 3rd year. I was sad when my last competition came because I was doing so well and knew there was so much more potential in me. The best part to end sophomore year was that we were able to have a competition in Beaver Dam. It was the best but it was also tough because I was attempting to squat 80 lbs for the first time and the first two attempts I went down too far and got stuck and then I fell forward, but on the third attempt everyone was cheering and I was able to easily get 80 lbs. I was excited but disappointed because I wanted more for how easy it was.

My opportunity finally came to play soccer. I was ready. It was unordinary but at least we got to play. We had to wear masks on the bus rides to the games, get our temps taken before getting on the bus and even wear a mask while playing on the field. It was an adjustment but we got used to it. The very first day of practice it was pouring rain outside and due to how many games we had and how very few practices we were going to be having our coaches decided to keep it. Everyone was freezing cold and our masks, coats, shorts, hair, cleats, etc. were soaking wet as soon as we stepped foot on the field.

As I previously stated I am a defender and with that comes risking your body to save the ball from going in the back of the net. Whether or not I like it, it is what it is. Since my first experience of getting hit I had done well at not getting hit again. Well, sophomore year I started getting hit again a couple times. One funny story in practice a girl named Riley was new to soccer and new to the team. It was her very first practice and she had the ball. We were in a small circle doing a drill and I was the defender in the middle, she went to kick the ball and when she kicked it, it hit me straight in the middle of my face on my nose. She felt so bad and asked me if I was okay and made the comment: "This is why I don't play soccer!" I was okay and we laughed it off and just kept on practicing. At the conclusion of my spring soccer season as I was transitioning into running for the summer again, I was noticing different changes in my body. My mindset was changing. I wasn't as "lean" and "muscular" as I had been during the summer and winter. I was starting to get agitated and didn't understand why. I hadn't changed what I was doing and I was trying to eat healthier. I got into my head a lot and questioned: "Why is it that I am eating healthier and exercising more and I am not as "lean and muscular" as I was before?" I still ran throughout the summer but this time it wasn't just for the joy and happiness I had felt coming out of it, I felt like I needed to exercise in order to get "fitter" and I wasn't finding the joy in it like I did before. I kept having the thoughts of "you can't take a day off or you'll feel like garbage and the best thing to feel even a little bit better is to go for a run" and "why am I running so slow, I didn't even run this slow when I first started running." I continued to eat salads and fruits at every meal and struggled to let myself eat anything besides that because I didn't want to "ruin" my body more. I struggled to allow myself to have a rest day where I maybe just went for a walk instead of a run or just took a day off. I didn't want my body to get any "worse" than I already thought it was. There were days where I would do anything just to make sure I had a run in after work no matter if it was blazing hot outside or not. I also wasn't feeling the muscle in my calves like I did before, making it harder for me to stay positive, so I decided that I would use the rest of my brother's membership and start Sports Advantage (the workout company that our school contracted with) for the rest of the summer to start incorporating both strength training and running.

To add onto the rough patch of my junior year, tennis started out a little rocky but improved as the year went on. At the very beginning of the season my coaches had paired me up with a new doubles partner who had very little experience with playing tennis. It was difficult at first to get used to the fact that I had to help her improve and learn the game while also trying to do my best in matches as well. Most of our matches at the beginning were a learning process for her but with work, dedication and perseverance we got out of those times and moved into better times. Sarah and I would work at tennis practice every day together and improve as a partnered team. There would be drills or tasks we would do that I would be able to give her tips on to help her improve. Throughout the season she significantly improved and by the end of the season we were winning most of our games together. Instead of feeling down about the games I was becoming more excited and happy with who I was playing with. Each match we became more of a team. A funny story about us playing together is that mostly every single match towards the end of the season ended in a tie breaker. We won most of those games but anytime that we got close we would look at each other and say "this is not ending in a tie breaker, we are ending it right here" and we did. We lifted each other up and gave each other positive words of encouragement when it was needed. Despite how hard the beginning of the season was she and I were both able to improve significantly and become better individuals and partners. She improved my game by improving her own game and mindset when on the court.

It was my favorite time of year again powerlifting time! Bringing the excitement from my 10th grade year I couldn't wait to get back to competing and lifting heavy weights, but it was nothing like my sophomore year. My mental thoughts were still a struggle and powerlifting became harder. I mentally thought that I had lost all of the muscle I gained in 2020 and I wasn't going to be as successful that year as I was before. The scale had said that I was at a lower weight but I wasn't as happy as I should have been. I compared myself to my old self during covid. I kept having the thoughts of "I ate pizza, pasta, macaroni, and frosted animal crackers everyday while I was running in 2020. Why was my body stronger and leaner then and now that I am eating healthy I feel like I am just gaining more fat and losing muscle?" I was longing for a gap in my thighs because I felt that if I didn't have one I would have more fat on my legs. I was constantly looking in the mirror and looking for that gap. However, when competing, I would have the strength to eat pasta the night before because carbs are good for your body, especially when you are going to lift. I would still only allow myself a little serving and no seconds because I was watching my weight to make my weight class and I thought if I ate seconds or too much pasta I would gain too much and be over my weight limit. Even though that wasn't the case, it was always in my head like that. After every meet I would "treat" myself and allow myself to eat an ice cream of some sort. My choice every time was a Ben and Jerry's small pint of ice cream.

That would be the only day that I would allow myself to eat "bad" and I would take that day and the day before my meet off of running. Once that one day was up I was back to eating "healthy" and running again. I was so cautious of my weight during that time and how I saw myself that I would even bring my own food to family holidays to make sure that I knew I was eating "healthy." I didn't really understand why I had these thoughts and it was hard to accept them.

Despite me trying to lift heavier weights I never seemed to succeed, it never felt as light and I couldn't complete it without losing balance. My first competition I was able to successfully squat 90 lbs but anything higher I was slightly too high in the squat for it to be good. It was frustrating but I continued to try and get stronger in practice. Similarly, in my deadlift I was able to get 115 lbs and it felt super light and easy but when I tried 120 lbs I was never successful. I would either slightly lose my balance, not get it all, or I would hinge slightly (use my knees to get it up) and so they wouldn't count it as a good lift. The same things kept recurring every meet throughout the season. I never knew why I couldn't just get 5 more lbs. I would try every meet to squat, deadlift and bench what I had my sophomore year and they were just feeling harder. Most people have huge PR's and increase weight by 5 lbs each year at least and I just felt stuck in a hole. One meet I was able to easily get 115 lbs for bench and the next I couldn't get it. It was tough mentally but I knew that it just meant that I had something to show next season.

I made myself a New Year's Resolution to have a more positive body image and allow myself to enjoy the foods that I want every once in a while. I also wanted to allow myself those rest days or walk days. When the new year started, I noticed that when I was running it was becoming more enjoyable. I saw my times go back to where they were before and I wasn't running because I needed to, I was running because I wanted to. I felt happier, more positive, and had better thoughts going through my head. I was starting to allow myself to eat ring bologna, pastas, chips, ice cream, etc. I didn't eat them all of the time but I was eating them in moderation.

Once my last meet officially ended I slowly transitioned into working with my soccer team. I worked out with Sports Advantage but I was attending open gyms when I could. I knew that if I wanted to play to my best ability that season that I would need to eat well and reward myself after. Between practices and eating I was starting to feel stronger, I felt changes happening in my body. I ate Clif Bars before my games so that I would have energy and I didn't have the thought, "I shouldn't eat this, this is too many calories." I ate it and went on with my game. I replayed two songs during the bus rides to the games and during warmups. They helped me mentally get in the right place to be the best me that I could be during my games. ("If You Believe" by Strive to Be, Patch Crowe, and "The Climb" by Miley Cyrus).

I play wearing my braces. Having them on has always helped me kick the ball better and have control and balance when moving around on the field and fighting for the ball when defending. Over the last year or so I started to realize that wearing my braces was affecting my ability to perform at my highest, specifically my speed and being capable of maneuvering the ball, so I wanted to look into some other alternative to my braces. Unfortunately, the options that were presented I thought would not be as beneficial and so I decided to stick with playing with my braces for the rest of the time. When the season officially started we met our new coach and from the beginning the program was different. She came in wanting to change the BD program around and she is starting to do that. Not only did we practice but we also did fitness days, and yoga days. It started out fun and then it got rough. Mentally it got really tough for me in games because of drama that was going on throughout the whole team. We tried to do team building activities for practice, meditation/yoga and during the time it seemed to work but other times when we stepped on the field the pressure was back. We all got through it and managed to stay together as a team and play and that is all that mattered. One tough moment that is still fresh to me is the game against Waunakee. We knew from the beginning that the game was going to be super tough and we were going to lose by a lot. What I didn't know was that it was going to be as bad as it was. We were losing by halftime 7-0. We got over to the sidelines and none of us were happy. We got in so much trouble especially as defenders for how the team was playing. Personally, I thought that the whole entire team was not playing their best and that the defenders were doing their best for what the players in front of us were doing. However that was not the case. Mentally, it made me down and I just wanted the game to end. Adding on to the bad vibe of the game, I also got a ball to the face. The whole time my timing was off and I was never in the right position for the ball so it always went around me, well except this one time.

This time the ball came straight for the left side/middle of my face. Once it hit my face the middle ref blew his whistle and the ref from the opposite side of the field yelled; "Hey number 3 are you ok" a little embarrassed I responded with yes and then was asked by my coach the same thing. Even though I was okay she had even taken me off the field for a little bit to make sure that I was really ok. It was a stinger for a few seconds but I was alright. At the end of the game the emotions came to me and I lost it. It was super hard because I already know that playing and keeping up is harder for me, so hearing that none of the defenders were contributing hurt me really bad because I felt that I was trying my best and wasn't getting any recognition for it.

I felt like I was growing out of many phases at the end of my soccer season and entering a new one because I was happier than I had previously been and during Easter when we got together to celebrate and have fun as a family I was still feeling happy and able to enjoy the food (and dessert) with my family and not feel guilty. Since my resolution was super important to me, I was committed to continuing it throughout the summer. I wanted to stay happier and not compare myself to anyone else or my past self and have a better summer than the year before. It was a struggle at times and there were moments where I had to remind myself that bodies change and I am stronger than I was before but I would say personally that I was able to enjoy this summer a lot more and worry less about eating super healthy. Too healthy does not mean better. My last year of business on the court was one to remember. I had a former tennis player from Beaver Dam work with me over the summer to continue my practice of tennis and I know that it helped me for this last season. I was able to try out for the varsity team and play a few matches on the varsity level. I didn't start playing with the same partner as last year but eventually we became partners again. Both of us girls had wanted to be partners again because we knew how each other played and we connected without needing to communicate where each of us were going to go on the court. She would always move to the back of the court and I was better at the net. Every opportunity we were partners. We were both so happy and she most importantly loved to be with me. She kept saying that I basically taught her tennis even though it was just her ability to practice and learn well. Every match we would get so excited and giddy during the match when we would make a shot that was either good or barely in.

There were also times where we would laugh at something that would happen or be upset for hitting the ball too hard/swinging our racket on a volley. We would enjoy playing together and having fun. There were games where we would be down and miraculously pull through with a win. One of those games being senior night. That night was one to remember. We played against Fort Atkinson at home and we were placed in 4 doubles. We started out not so great and were down 2-0 against a team that we knew in our heads we shouldn't have been down to. We made some silly mistakes that cost us those first two points. Through our determination and fight we were able to turn it around and get back into the game. We were able to get us to 2-2 and then it went to 6-3 and we won the match 9-7 in a tie breaker. Both Sarah and I knew that it was not going to end with us losing and so we gave everything we had to get back into that game. Playing in a match like that for my senior year was so special and it was amazing that we were able to get a win off it too.

Just when you think all things are good and going your way, something seriously unexpected can happen. One normal Saturday morning I was eating breakfast and getting ready to leave for my tennis matches. All of a sudden I felt this sharp pain shoot to my right and travel through my side and land in my right kidney. It was definitely something I had never felt before. At first it was super painful but it subsided quickly to just a little discomfort. I still managed to get ready to go to the bus for my matches. The ride there wasn't painful. During the first match that day it had bothered me but I was still able to move around the court and be pretty active and consistent in the match. Once that first game was over we had a break and the pain in my kidney had stayed the same. I got a little stiff from sitting for long periods but otherwise I felt the same minimal discomfort. My mom and I were thankful that it wasn't progressing worse. About an hour later, our second match had started and that was when things started to get worse. Immediately, during warmups I could not move around the court like normal. Anytime I would try to make an effort to run, my body would not want to do it. I wasn't really in the game. Whenever I would run across to hit the ball or any type of movement, my kidney would bring discomfort and I wouldn't be able to sprint for the ball or get in position quick enough to hit the ball accurately. Every time I would try to serve, it was hard to focus. My hands were sweaty even when my body was at normal temperature. It just wasn't a very good game for me. This made it difficult for my partner as well. We unfortunately lost that match and so we were done for the day.

Once my last tennis match was over, my mom and the coach (who is a nurse and has known me basically my whole life) said that they thought it would be a good idea to go to Urgent Care in Beaver Dam and get checked out. Agreeingly, we headed home and I was pretty tired. My back/kidney were uncomfortable on my right side when I walked at a normal pace or any faster, so I would walk slower but otherwise I felt normal. It didn't hurt to sit, breathe, etc. We arrived at the urgent care and they had gotten us into a room and gave me a warm blanket to cover up in. They decided to run tests to check for an infection or to rule it out. Shortly after I had gotten back in the room they started me on fluids for hydration to relieve some pain. At this point I was so cold but warm to the touch which probably meant I had a fever. What felt like 3 hours later, the results came back that there was an air bubble in my kidney. Since they had never really seen that before, they decided to talk with my doctors at the UW Hospital in Madison. We were told the air bubble would go away on its own in a day or two. They also made sure that they had done everything at the time they could before sending me home. All I wanted to do was go home but all of this was taking a long time.

After 3 ½ hours of being there, and just as I was about to be released, someone came in and drew some more blood. They wanted to make sure there weren't any infections in my blood. For how exciting it was to go home, it was definitely a downward spiral. When I got home, I started to shiver and shake uncontrollably. I took a hot bath to warm myself up and then I layed in bed. My mom tried so hard to get me to eat dinner because I hadn't really eaten anything all day but I didn't have an appetite. All I wanted to do was sleep (something that didn't take any effort). So I didn't eat and layed down and slept all night until mid-morning. Unfortunately, the next morning I woke up and my head still felt heavy. I was out of it and just not feeling the greatest. My back was sore but not really in any discomfort like the day before. I tried to eat some eggs for breakfast but they tasted kind of bland, not something I was interested in eating and so I only had a little bit. My parents had their camp volunteer brunch that morning too and I really wanted to go.

As my mom and I started getting ready to go, my mom got a call from the doctors in Urgent Care saying that the results from the blood work were positive and that I had an infection in my blood. They didn't specify at that time what it was but they advised that I be taken care of at UW Madison Children's Hospital since the doctors there knew me and my birth defect. So being my crazy self, I wanted to go to the brunch first and then go to the hospital (At this point though too I wasn't bad and I felt just tired and thought it would go away). About a couple minutes after they called the first time, they called again and confirmed with us that it was E Coli in my blood. Thankful that my parents let me, we went to the brunch together. I still walked slowly and was not 100% functioning like I wanted to be but I enjoyed my time and was glad that I had gone and saw some of my camping friends. Then we headed out to the hospital where things got worse before they got better. The whole drive to the hospital I could tell I was warm to the touch but felt cold. I had a sweatshirt on and a blanket over me but I was still a little cold and my head felt so heavy that I couldn't focus all the way. We arrived at the ER in Madison and got through security, my mom checked me in and then they had taken my vitals. They asked me what had brought me in, checked my pulse in my finger, my blood pressure, and my temperature which had been at 103. I was completely tired, cold, and my head felt super heavy the whole time while waiting and all I wanted to do was rest my head on something. Once my name was called a nurse took me to a small room where he gave me some Tylenol right away to help with my high fever and gave me some IV fluid antibiotics to get me feeling better as soon as possible.

During this process, a doctor came in and explained to my parents what was going to happen later on in the day, and the next couple days, and what could have possibly caused all of this to happen to begin with. Hooked up to my IV antibiotics, they put me back out in the waiting room where I waited for a room to be ready. While waiting to go back to a temporary room I dozed in and out of sleep and just tried to stay as warm as I could. As we were waiting I could tell that the fluids and medicine were working because my body started to get less cold and I could sit without my blanket on my legs and not wear my sweatshirt. Approximately 15 minutes after sitting there with my fluids someone came in and got me and walked me to a room that I was temporarily in until they had an overnight room ready for me to transfer to. Right away they got me hooked up to the heart monitors and other monitors on my body and watched my fever closely. The first time they had checked my temperature after the Tylenol it had gone down slightly. Doctors after doctors came in to get the rundown of what was going on with me and to talk about what they had gotten from Beaver Dam Urgent Care.

Some nurses came in to get some blood and others came in to give me ibuprofen. My fever continued to drop and I started to feel slightly better.

After waiting for 4 hours, a lot of tv watching and talking later, we were finally transferred upstairs where I was for 2 nights and 3 days. To get upstairs they brought a wheelchair and wheeled me up. We got upstairs and there were nurses that checked my vitals again and got me ready for my stay. They hooked me up to my monitors again and got the IV fluid antibiotics going and I was just able to relax and order dinner for the night. When I got dinner I had a great appetite and was able to enjoy it. The rest of the night I just layed in the bed, rested, and watched tv. Before going to bed the nurse had also informed us that she would come in every 4 hours to check my vitals and try to not wake me up. The first night, I had woken up when she came in because she needed to give me more ibuprofen. Then she came back at 4 am and checked my vitals again. Walking from the bed to the bathroom and back to the bed the first night was rough in itself. I was so unevenly balanced that I had to walk slowly to stay stable.

The next morning while I was asleep, a group of doctors and nurses had come in and talked to my mom about what the day would hold. They said that there would be an MRI scheduled for me that would help determine where the infection came from and what the next steps were to getting me healed and home. That Monday morning was a good morning. I had a minimal heavy head but my body temperature was normal and I hadn't felt cold. Rightbefore they were supposed to come get me for my MRI, things started to go backwards again and I got super cold but felt warm and my head was massively heavy. It would hurt to turn my head in any direction. Thankfully, when they came to transport me, they had a wheelchair and a warm blanket. So I didn't have to walk anywhere but from my bed to the wheelchair. We arrived at the MRI room and they started the tests. The MRI technician told me that she would tell me when I needed to hold my breath. Usually, when I am in there it isn't too bad and I am able to focus and be calm. With everything that was happening, I was unable to focus and the only thing that made it easier for me was to close my eyes.

Holding my breath many times for about 20 seconds each time was a struggle.

Twenty minutes later we were done and I was exhausted and hurting. I just wanted to get back up to the room. Once we arrived back at the room, I fell asleep and didn't wake up until later that night.

Unfortunately when I woke up my fever was back. I got some ibuprofen and ate dinner that my dad had brought me. Shortly after, I had started to feel the best I had in two days. I was able to walk to the bathroom without feeling uneven and my head was completely fine and I was able to turn it without hurting. Monday night I was still in the hospital being monitored but feeling a lot better. Doctors had come in and talked about the results of the MRI. They had confirmed that it had started out as an infection that went untreated, then went to my kidneys and spread to my blood. Meanwhile this whole time I hadn't had any symptoms at all.

Same thing happened Monday night as Sunday night, a doctor came in to check on me. Tuesday morning rolled around and I was still sleeping in until at least early to mid-morning and so there was a doctor that had come in and talked to my mom about what would happen that day as well. Most of the morning I just relaxed and watched tv, did some studying for tests that were supposed to be in the next day or two, and talked to some family members who were concerned about me. Then, around later morning into afternoon, the team of doctors came in and gave us the plan. They said the MRI had shown them where the infection had come from and they were able to diagnose a specific pill for me that I would need to take at home to continue my recovery. They mentioned that my fever had stayed down for a while so, as long as my fever would stay down, I was able to go home later that day, with restrictions on working out and playing tennis. About two hours later my doctor came in and told me that my fever hadn't spiked in a while and I was cleared to go home after one more bag of fluids. They gave me one last bag of fluids, checked my vitals, and removed all the needles and IVs. I was given a flu shot and I was walking myself out of the hospital.

I was still not feeling 100%. Even though the way home was still rough, I was able to get some sleep. I woke up the next morning for school and I was back to feeling good. I went to a full day of school and felt like myself. Then I went to tennis practice and did all of the things that we normally do but took things slower and was more aware and cautious but still felt alive, like I could do it forever. It was a complete shock to me how quickly I was able to turn around. The next morning, I went back to work out where I took things light and slow. It was tougher on my body but it still felt good that I was able to get back to working out and moving my body because it had been at least 5 days since I had last had some movement. The next 11 days, I took my antibiotics twice a day to continue my recovery process. A month later I went for a checkup to make sure my kidneys were good and the results came back that my kidneys are healthy.

This experience was difficult, but it made me learn that you need to have a strong mindset for happiness. Progress won't be linear, but you need to enjoy the journey. It'll be tough but the ones who don't give up show the most strength. If it doesn't challenge you, it won't change you.

Fast forward, and we get to our last matches and my last match as a Beaver Dam tennis player. I am all rested and excited to end my career strong. We had to split up playing matches in two days. As a senior, I got to choose which place I wanted to go and I had chosen Stoughton. We loaded up in the team vans and drove to Stoughton where I was paired up with a freshman who was also new at tennis but had really started to improve since the beginning of the year. She and I were able to work together and figure out our strengths. I was able to give her some tips that helped us communicate and know when the other was supposed to get the ball. This made my last tennis match one that I could have never pictured, and the best part is that we ended on a win. As I am writing this, I am in the middle of my last powerlifting season. I am loving it and working towards PR's (personal records) and getting stronger each and every day and although soccer is in the spring, I have enjoyed playing with most of the same teammates since 5th grade. They have all been supportive and see me as a leader, teammate, and a soccer player who is trying her best. As well as all my coaches that I have had. Sports has given me so much that I didn't know I could have.

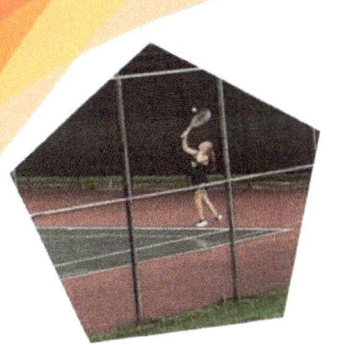

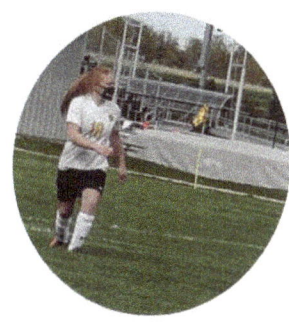

Sophomore Year

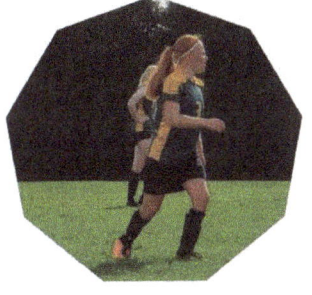

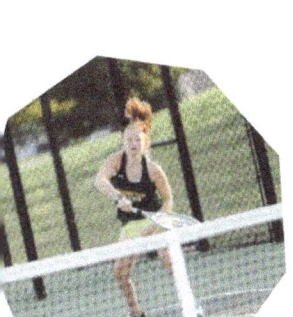

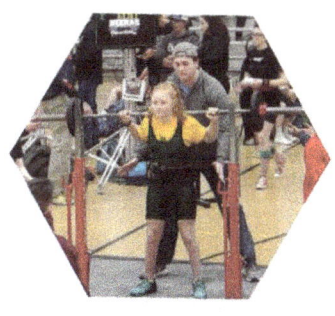

Junior Year

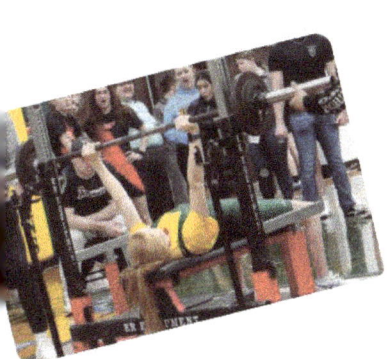

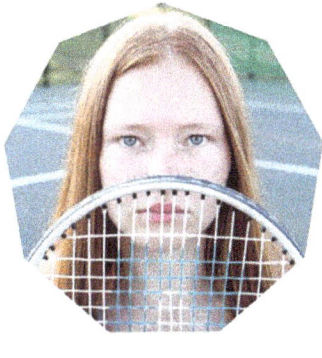

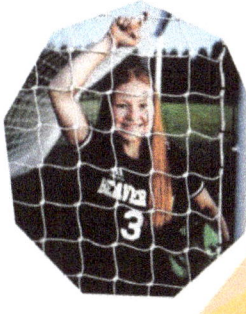

Senior Year

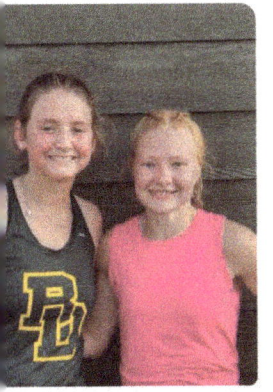

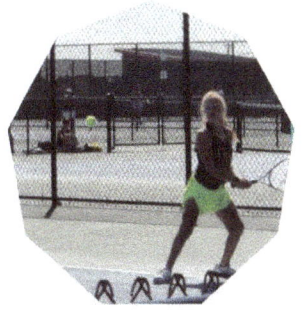

Friends

"A friend is one who overlooks your broken fence and admires the flowers in your garden."

Through school, sports, and clubs I have been able to find and meet many new friends, some that I still have and some that have gone on a different path, that have helped shape me into the person I am today, but my lifelong friendships began when I was in Daycare. At 12 weeks old when I went into daycare for the first time, I didn't know I would come out with some friends that I still have to this day. Abbey, Lauren, and Emma were the first girls that I met and became friends with. We met in the baby room at Daycare. We played together all the time on the playground and became such good friends right away. Abbey and I always laugh because her last name is long and super hard for many people to pronounce and so we joke and say that when we were able to speak I would say my friend: Abbey Kasuboski (I would pronounce it as Ka-bow-ski). In 4K we started to have a lot of sleepovers and playdates which allowed us to create so many fun memories as little kids.

When the time came to go off to elementary school, we all went to South Beaver Dam and just like any transition from one school to the next, you add more kids to the class so the size goes from 15 to 25 or 30 kids. Having the door open to so many more people who could become a next friend can be scary especially when you are starting Kindergarten and like me with braces, but it was a positive experience and one that I will be grateful for, for the rest of my life. I not only stayed friends with Abbey, Lauren, and Emma but I also gained many new ones, both boys and girls. I was able to meet Kendra, Nathan, Mitchell, Luis, Hailey, Lindsey, Ariana, Shayla, Karla, Kaleigh, and Kirsten, to name a few.

Every day at recess Abbey, Kendra, Nathan and I would either go to the back corner of the yard where there were trees and just have a fun time or we would play basketball, swing on the swings, play four square and, last but definitely not least, play tetherball. When we would go to the back corner we stayed back there the whole time until we were whistled to come back in and would try not to get seen by anybody. We succeed most of the time. For a short while, tetherball was super fun and something we would consistently play. No matter what I wanted to do or play I always had friends that I was able to hang out with that made it fun for both of us.

The days that I didn't hang out with them I hung out with one of my friends at the time, Hailey, on the monkey bars. We would hang upside down, move across them or we would climb up into them and get to the very top and sit. It was a new thing we were all trying to master.

Sadly, our hobbies started to change once we were transitioning into middle school and some of my friends had left and went to a different middle school, but most of my friends that I had in elementary school were still my friends. I had classes where I met new friends, for example in my Reading class I met a girl, Hailey, who was very nice and very smart who ended up becoming one of my friends that I enjoyed talking to in middle school. She saw me as smart, funny, pretty, kind and not someone who was different. There were also times that my other friends had other friend groups and hung out with them as well but overall, I stuck with the same 5 friends that I had in elementary school. We definitely had our disagreements, fights, arguments but we were always there for each other. We sat at lunch together and had our designated spot that fit all of us and that was it. We always ate together no matter what. Some days we hung out outside for our "recess" time because it was all the time we would have together because we all didn't have the same classes.

Now being in high school has made it different. We all have mostly different classes and lunches and it has made it difficult to have time to see and hang out with my friends. My freshmen year I was fortunate because I had 3 classes with my friend Kendra from Kindergarten. We were able to walk to our classes together, have lunch together, and sit next to each other in class. Having her in a lot of my classes made it easier for me to transition to a bigger setting and it gave me the confidence to know that there was someone with me that accepted me. Similarly, Kaleigh and I had a locker right across from each other and Abbey's was just down the hall a little bit so every morning we would meet at someone's locker before class started and Abbey and I would walk to class together since she and I had English. Even though Nathan, Mitchell and Kaleigh weren't in any of my classes I was still able to hang out with them and see them throughout the day and after school.

The next couple years of high school I had some classes with Abbey, Kendra, Nathan, Kaleigh, or Jordyn, but the times when we really got to hang out would be on the weekends or nights after school. Our times spent doing something together would be during girl scouts, service opportunities, summer get togethers and a random weekend. They have made my life growing up so special.

With all the fun we have had at school, my friends and I have hung out a lot on the weekends and during the summer and have had so much fun right from the start.

I met Nathan before school started when I had moved from my original neighborhood to the one I live in now. We became and are still across the street neighbors. It was a recurrence for Nathan and his brother to come over on the weekends, days off of school and in the summer to go swimming and play on the slip n slide that we laid out in our yard. Most times it would be the store bought one but a couple times we made our own with a tarp, water from the hose, and dawn dish soap. As little kids we took advantage of the dish soap and most of the time soaked the slip n slide with it to make it as slippery as possible. Once the slip n slide was coded we would race to see who could go down the farthest and fastest and then there would be times where we would try to climb back up the Slip & Slide and see who could get back all the way to the top. We would be laughing and playing for hours every day in the summertime and weekends when it was warm out. Days when we didn't want to go swimming in the pool or slide down the slip n slide all four of us would play football or when we were really young we would ride bikes. Most of the time it would be my brother and I vs. Griffin and Nathan.

During high school we were also lucky to have the opportunity to participate in powerlifting together for one year. We worked out together every day and motivated and pushed each other to continue to get stronger. We would laugh at each other and he would always call me "Shoulders" because of my jacked shoulders that I had.

Abbey and I did everything from the beginning together. We grew up playing on the same soccer team for a couple of years together. Abbey was the goalie and I was one of the defenders for our team. Our moms became friends from the beginning so we spent a lot of time talking about our games and it was something that was fun for all of us. Over the couple of years playing together our friendship grew not only off the field but also on the field. We enjoyed playing together so much. It made my first couple of early years in a sport that much more fun and memorable. She has said that she looked at me and knew that if I was able to do it that she would also be able to do it. She channeled her inner "You only live once" motto that I say and live by. We had many weekend nights where we slept over, played, and swam together. Every birthday party Abbey had was something with a sleep over and one that I remember specifically we made macaroni and cheese and ate it with hot dogs, but instead of just doing that we decided to add a twist and so we decided we wanted to try putting syrup on it and so we did. I will say it wasn't bad but also not something I would have regularly. We have gone through 12 years of girl scouts together and gone on many trips, adventures and activities. She joined 1 year into me already being into it but otherwise we have gone through every event, challenge, and fun moment together. She is always someone that I look to for advice, encouragement and over all what life has to offer. She is one of the best people I spend my spare time with and I know that we can always have a laugh together no matter what. She makes me feel so confident and worthy and she assures me that I am buff.

Along with Abbey, I have also been fortunate to meet Jordyn through girl scouts. Her mom has been my leader for girl scouts and so many of our memories together are through girl scouts. From the very first day of walking into girl scouts she has been another one that I can automatically feel connected and in a laughy mood with. She has accepted me and given me an example of what it means to be independent, strong and not take no for an answer. Every girl scout event or school activity that we have encountered together has been amazing and there has always been laughs along the way. She has always been so inviting and willing to bring people in for events with school, her birthday, and girl scouts and doesn't like to exclude anyone. Every birthday party for at least the last 5 years she has invited me and we have done some amazing, fun things. They provide everything for us to make me and the rest of her friends feel welcome and inviting. Likewise, for homecoming this past year, a couple of her friends, Kendra, and I were able to hang out before the dance. We ate pizza, got ready together, and then had an after-party at her house. It was fun and super kind of her to be so inviting. Last but not least, Abbey and I were able to spend a night with her and Tammy and Jen to see the Trans-Siberian Orchestra. The night was amazing and definitely full of laughs thanks to the ability to hang out with all of those girls.

The last member of the troop that I have been friends with from the beginning is Kendra. She and I have been able to see each other and interact a lot more in high school during class time than I have with my other friends. Her, Abbey, and I would have many sleepovers for her birthday party where we would play games in her basement and eat cheesecake for dessert.

Funny enough, it was at her house that I realized I didn't like avocados. My most favorite memory at her birthday parties was when we would hand out our presents to her and she would open them. Mostly every present I got her would be a new game so we would spend the rest of the night playing the new games and having fun while laughing. My favorite game that I got her one year was Tick Tock Boom. You have three letters on a card, and you have a die that says tick, tock or boom. Whatever you roll indicates where in a word those three letters must be placed. Tick means at the beginning; Tock means at the end and Boom means anywhere in the word. After you start there is a bomb that is making noise and you try to not have the bomb go off on your turn.

It was super funny and we all had a great time because it was very hard for her and Abbey to come up with words and it didn't seem too hard for me. I enjoyed it so much I got it for me at my house.

Besides birthday parties and girl scouts, we have been able to volunteer and help at places together serving others and it has been a lot of fun. She is a very smart, kind, incredible person with a great heart and someone I know that I can go to for advice when I need it. I can go to her if I need something, and she will have a logical answer. I am very grateful that she sees me as I am and not what I look like.

Kaleigh Schweitzer. A friend of mine that feels like we have been on a roller coaster together. We met in elementary school, and we have been friends ever since. We have had many good memories together and some that show just how true our friendship is together. Not every friendship that you encounter in your life is going to go smoothly but the ones that work and that are meant to work always come through the hard and find the light. We always got along in elementary school, and we were the best of friends. We lived across a busier road in the subdivisions across the street, so it was like a 2 minute drive from each other. Anytime she had a Halloween party I was invited, and we had a great time. Their family was very inviting. We had multiple sleepovers just the two of us and I had a blast. My most favorite sleepover to date was when she invited me to go to her church and do games and sleep with her there. We played games and had food all night long.

Every year our neighborhoods do a trick or treating together and when we were younger and less busy all of us friends, Abbey, Nathan, Kendra, Kaleigh, Mitchell, and I would go out together and get candy from the houses and then go back to someone's house and dump out all our candy and play in the yard and at dark play Ghost in the Graveyard. It was really fun.

Then in Middle School some things happened but we were able to reconcile our friendship. Our friendship became the best it had ever been. Then when we got the opportunity to be locker neighbors across the hall, which was fun. But when covid happened she decided to stay virtual for a couple of years and so we never really got to see each other. We still communicated over Snapchat but that was it. We hadn't had anymore sleepovers, hangouts, etc.

When the opportunity came, I took advantage of it. For our junior prom I asked her if she wanted to come with Kendra and I because we hadn't hung out or seen each other for a long time and I thought it would be fun. Her and Kendra both came over to get ready and take pictures and then we all went to dinner together. I will remember that and be thankful that we were able to become friends again and reconnect after some time down. She is an amazing girl with a big heart.

I have realized over the years that I don't need a lot of friends in my life for me to feel worthy and accepted. For me the only friends I need and want are the ones that I have had from the very beginning that know who I am from the inside not the out. I know that there may be a lot of kids who have a condition or a disability that may get mistreated by others but those are the people who aren't worth your time. The true friends that I have don't care about my spina bifida, rather they are proud, astonished, and grateful for what I have given to them, and I am grateful for what they have given to me. They uplift me and encourage me to go after my dreams and know that I can do anything in my life that I want to.

Whether I looked silly as a little girl who came in with braces on my legs, all they saw in me was my personality and drive. They wanted to be my friend and they didn't seem to care that I was "different" from them. We all didn't have the same friend groups but the majority of us went to each other's birthday parties, hung out at each other's house on the weekends, and went swimming or did different things.

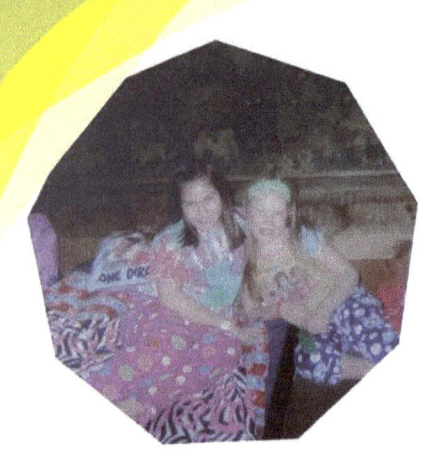

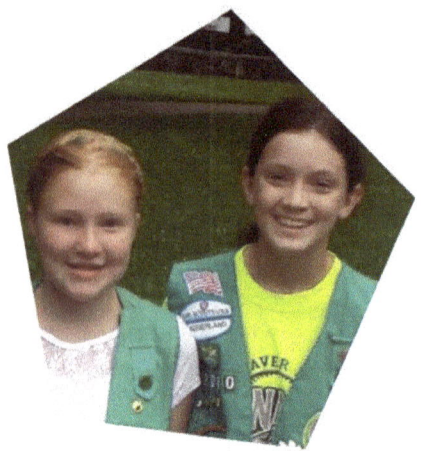

Kendra and I at the Milwaukee Muesum for a Girl Scout sleepover. We slept in front of the pigs.

Abbey and I at a Girl Scout ceremony as Juniors bridging to Cadettes.

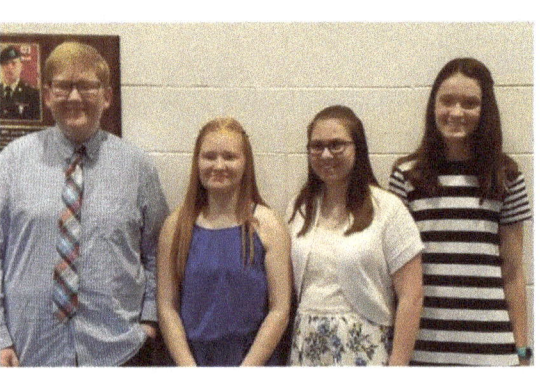

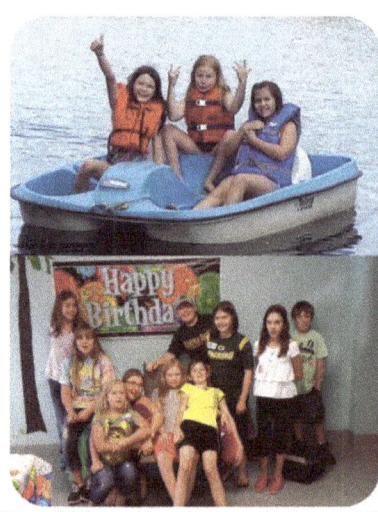

Nathan, Me, Kendra, Abbey at our 8th grade graduation.

Top: Abbey, Kendra, and me paddl boating at Willow Mill Campground Bottom: Birthday party at Animar with my friends from school.

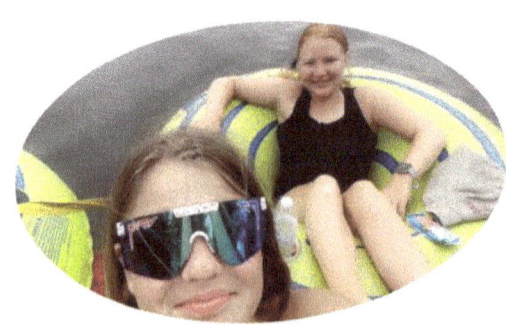

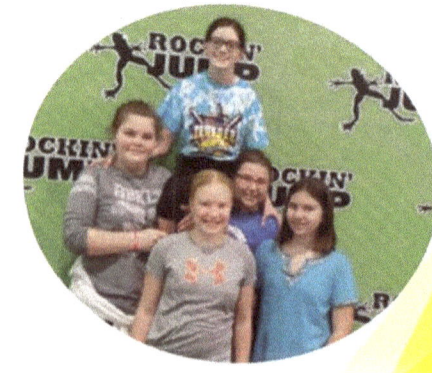

My Friend Olivia and I tubing at Point Bluff with her family and friends.

Birthday party destination: Rockin' Jump.

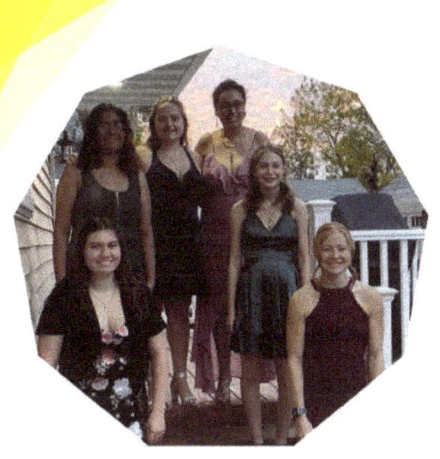

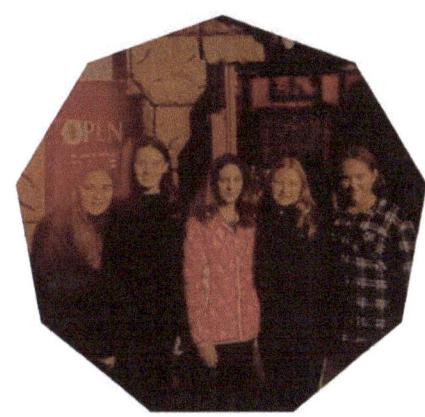

First haunted house experience for me: Halloween party Kaleigh hosted.

Homecoming 2022: (Top to Bottom): Lizet, Jordyn, Shayla, McKenzie, Kendra, and Me.

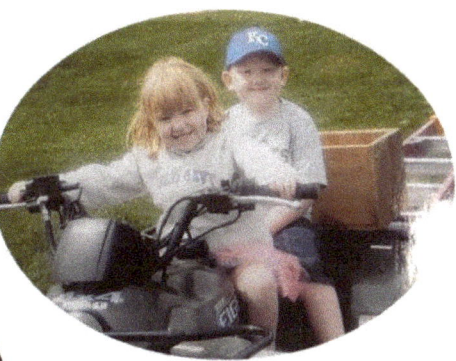

Nathan and I on a four wheeler.

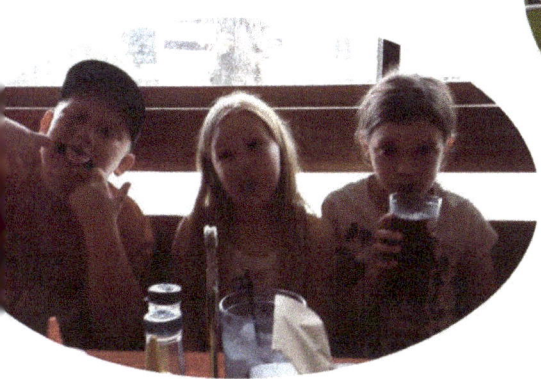

Nathan, Me and Abbey being our crazy selves.

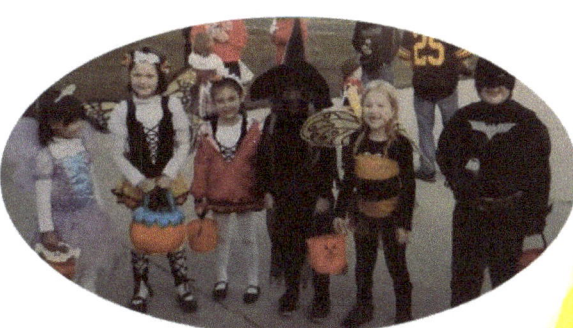

Trick or Treating in Zimmerman and Hillview Dr.

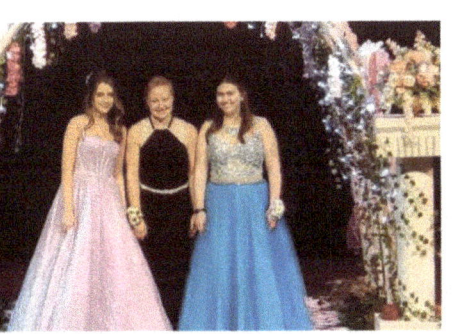

Kaleigh, Me and Kendra at prom 2022.

Love what you do, do it with Passion

If you love to do something you continue to do it for multiple years until you are no longer eligible. When I was in Kindergarten, I started Girl Scouts. It has given me the ability to grow, learn and develop skills that show others that no matter what the circumstances, you can accomplish anything and do it with passion. As you age you become a higher-level girl scout. The levels in order are **Daisy, Brownie, Junior, Cadette, Senior, Ambassador.** I was able to join and start as a daisy. Each level gives you the ability to have different experiences and opportunities that you can partake in that are fun. As a younger girl scout you aren't able to decide what you do, it is mostly up to the leaders to decide what activities you are going to do and places you are going to visit. My leaders had given us the opportunities to do corn mazes, horseback riding, make and deliver valentines to the elderly, set up a cookie booth, etc. The very first time that we went horseback riding we went single file and followed a path. Since most of us were doing it for the first time, we weren't allowed to trot.

The next couple times that we decided we wanted to go horseback riding we went to the same place and were able to trot and run a little bit, but it was still single file.

Instead of driving back home we made the choice to stay in the little houses that were on the property. We slept on wooden slab bunk beds and although no one else was comfy I was not too bad. For both times my horse's name was Speed Bump and he was super old and for sure fit his name. The very first time I had him he held up the group a lot but made up for the second time around when he went a little faster.

We have had several sleepover parties at the girl scout house. Watching movies and doing different activities. One of the sleepover activities that we have done together that I will never forget is doing a blindfold makeup challenge. It was the worst experience of my life. I was wearing braces on my teeth and my partner was not very good at applying makeup while not being able to see and by the end I had make up in my braces that took a while to come off.

Sleepovers don't always have to be in a house or tent/camper, they can be anywhere but what I wasn't expecting was to sleep somewhere like this. Our troop had the opportunity to sleep at the Milwaukee Museum by the exhibits. It was very interesting but it was cool at the same time. Anywhere we looked we saw some type of exhibit thing whether it was a stuffed animal, person, artifact, etc. Kendra and I both slept next to each other under the pigs. We got used to it and survived a night at the museum.

As a junior girl scout we started to really get involved and started making and planning events with our leaders. One of them was taking one of our family members with us to sew our Girl Scout vests together at Nancy's Notions. I chose my grandma because she has sewn her whole life and is the one who put all the patches on my vests throughout the years. It was a nice experience and helpful that I had someone with me that knew how to work a machine like that.

The other great opportunity you get as a junior girl scout is the opportunity to be involved and participate in a Junior Jamboree, which our troop joined in 2015. We were 10 years old. The Junior Jamboree consists of events that require your arms, legs, brain, and your whole body.

The first event that we always did was the Tug of War; my favorite. My arm strength that I developed through swimming and other activities was crucial for the tug of war and allowed me to be in the back as the anchor. My teammates and I were dominant at the event every year. We won and got the trophy for it! Additionally, there was also an event that required us to wear flip flops, glasses and clothes while being in the water. It was a race to see who could swim down and back and then remove the clothes you had on over your swimming suit while still being in the water. There were 4 members on a team. The first person was the lucky one because the clothes were dry when you first put them on. The key thing was that you had to take the clothes off right side up. They couldn't be inside out. I struggle with moving my toes so I hadn't always done that event, but it was the last year for us to be eligible for this, so I was committed to trying my hardest to help our team get a result. Knowing it was going to be harder for me to wear the flip flops in the water, keep them on, and walk across the pool that gradually got deeper, I had to adjust to my abilities and figure out a different way to get across. I improvised and had my foot go through the loop of the sandal instead of where they were supposed to. This worked and I was able to help my team win a ribbon for first place! My troop encouraged and uplifted me and told me that no matter how I had to, I could do it!

Continuing with the water events came the hand paddling canoe race. The hand paddling canoe race consists of 3 people in a canoe. When the race begins, each person paddles with their hands as fast as they can. The people who paddle the canoe in the fastest amount of time wins. Abbey, Hannah, and I were all in a canoe together when the time began, I started to paddle as fast as I could and tried to move us along but instead I was scooping the water and apparently splashing Abbey behind me and getting water in her face while also putting water in the canoe. Whoopsie! It didn't matter though because we won a ribbon.

Other events throughout the day included: water carry, balloon toss, balancing on a raft in the water, tied three-legged race, and geocaching.

To finish off the day they had an event called The Relay Race. Four people working individually but all timed together as a team. Someone does trivia, someone walks with a book on their head, and someone guides someone else who is blind folded. My role was to do the trivia because the group thought I was the smartest one and knew the most information.

As juniors, cadettes, seniors, and ambassadors we started getting into something that has really turned into something that I think we all enjoy doing. Teaching badges of our choice to our group. My very first badge that I taught was called New Cuisines. It involved learning how to cook and make food and it was delicious. We made pizza pocket like things, and yogurt parfaits. A few more of my badges included Field Day, Locavore, Simple Meals, Night Owl, and Cross-Training. My most recent badge that I taught was Coaching. I was able to teach Kendra, Jordyn, and Jen, tennis skills and components required to be successful in both tennis and in any sport in general. In addition, we watched a video that taught us what it takes to be a successful person/coach and how motivation and positivity takes a team a long way. Finally, they learned how proper warmups and cooldowns are essential for getting your body ready for your sport or activity.

Other badges that I have learned are Car Care, Art, First Aid, Woodworking, Trees, etc. I feel that they are not only a learning opportunity for all of us but we also have fun with them.

One of my favorite things about becoming an older girl scout is the fun we have gotten to have.

One of our very first big trips was to Chicago but this was not like any of the other ones that we went on later. We didn't drive to Chicago; we took the Amtrak train from Columbus. We were so excited to be going on a train for the first time together. We had arrived at the train station as a troop and we waited with excitement and unlike the previous experience I had with my family our train arrived on time. All of us boarded the train and we found our seats. Once settled and going we enjoyed the ride. We rode through the morning and got there in the afternoon. In Chicago we settled into our hotel and walked to Millennium Park to take pictures, see the bean and all the cool things around the park. After the park we enjoyed some ice cream and played games at our hotel. We had so many things planned that we were hoping to have good weather but we were unlucky, but that didn't prevent us from having fun still. We visited the Navy Pier, shopped around, and enjoyed a ride on the ferris wheel. We also rode on the double decker bus in the rain and decided to go on the top with our rain ponchos on. It was a rainy ride and we were the only ones up top but we enjoyed getting information about Chicago and seeing around the city. The whole trip was rainy and cold and not the best experience for us but our plans remained the same. We enjoyed a super cool lunch at the Rainforest Cafe and a trip to Willis Tower. On our last day we reserved tickets to go to the top and see the views. Unfortunately, the day we went it was foggy, cloudy and we couldn't see anything when we looked out or down, but we walked around the top and looked at different information stands they had. It was scary to walk out on the little platforms with clear glass around you and clear glass underneath you, but we were brave enough to look down and see nothing but the building underneath us because of the fog. It was disappointing to not get the weather we wanted on the trip but it wasn't our first trip that was like that.

Junior Jamboree: Our troop with
ribbons, as well as us competing in the tug
of war and obstacle course.

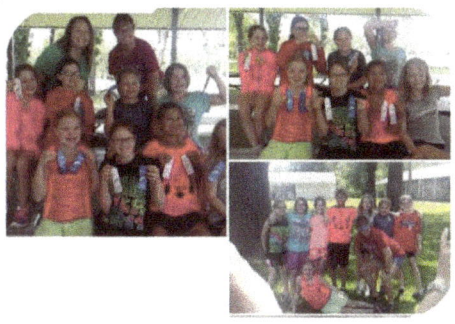
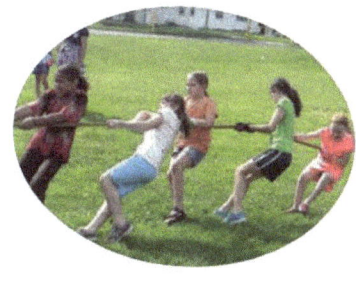

Door County: a trip planned by Abbey where we were able
to go cliff jumping, hiking, etc.
Our surprise trip for the leaders to the Dells: Cheese Ball
Heads, and Wizard Quest.

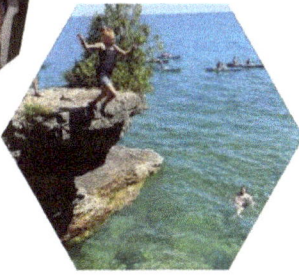
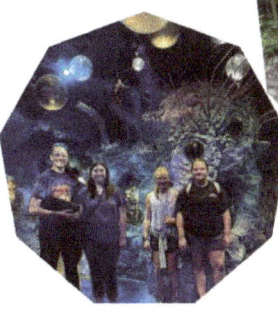

Three of our window painting designs.
We picked them to resemble our
events throughout Girl Scouts and
then finally us moving on.

Left & top: St. Vincent Food
Pantry; Bottom: Police
Department.

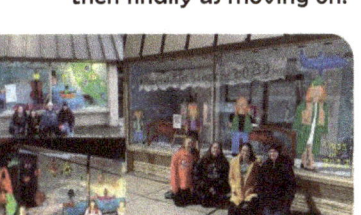
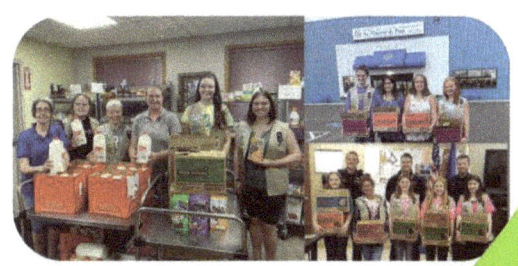

In 2019 my troop and I planned a kayaking trip to the Apostle Islands. If you don't know anything about it, it consists of multiple small islands spread out over a large area and the water is freezing cold. For safety purposes we had to take a "tip test", as they called it, so you knew what to do if you and your partner were to tip over in your kayak and to prevent hypothermia, we wore wetsuits. My kayak partner, Zoe, and I did the tip test together. It was the scariest moment in my life. We paddled from shore to our spot and were instructed to grab the side of our covering of our kayak or skirt, bring our hands to the front, and pull it off as we flipped the kayak.

Well, that is not as easy as it sounds! I was unsuccessful in getting the skirt off when we flipped, so I hung upside down in the water, panicking, because the skirt wasn't off and the kayak was on top of me. I shortly after figured out that I could possibly try to squirm my way out and thankfully that worked. Once Zoe and I were both above water, we flipped our kayak right way up and had to lift ourselves back in. Since my skirt was still attached to the kayak, the guide had me try to get back into the seat with it on. It worked! Once each tandem team completed the test, we were ready to go to our first island. We loaded all our food, sleeping items, clothes, etc. into waterproof bags and loaded it in our kayaks.

As we started to paddle out to our first island it took some time to get used to but once we got the hang of it, we did well. Our guides told us that kayaking on Lake Superior required strength from not only your arms but also your core. The more I used my core to paddle the less tired my arms became. After two hours of paddling, and many views of open water later, we made it to our first island.

The next step was to unload the kayaks and get the camp set up. To be efficient and effective everyone had a specific job that they were required to do each night. This included getting wood and building a fire, setting up tents, making meals, and cleaning up meals. It consistently changed who was doing what job.

To get wood for the fire, two people had to walk down the path searching for pieces that were already cut and dry. It was difficult because a lot of the pieces we found were wet or not cut up. Once wood was found we got the fire going. While the fire was getting started a couple other people were setting up the tents for everyone and we four girls figured out where we were going to sleep inside the tent. After that we ate the food that was prepared for us and got ready for a good night's sleep from a long day of paddling by putting all our vibrant smelling things in a box away from all of our tents to prevent attracting bears to our tent.

The next morning things changed. Our guides told us that the weather was going to worsen, and we needed to leave early for the mainland. If we wanted to stay, we would be stuck on the next island we were supposed to go to for at least 5 days (It was Monday and we would be stuck until Friday). So, we decided that we would go back, cutting our trip short. We quickly packed, loaded the kayaks, and set out back to the mainland. This time the guides had switched up the pairing and thought that it was better that Jordyn and I go together. The guides were right, once Jordyn and I focused on our task, we were leaders of the pack. We were called the "dream team" because apparently, we were so in sync with each other.

Closer and closer to shore, the clouds started to roll in, the waves started picking up and some of the time our kayaks were pointing up in the front. The worst came as soon as we got to the landing spot. We loaded the kayaks onto the bus as the rain was coming down on us and by the time we were undressed from our wetsuits and back in our regular clothes, it was pouring outside. We all said that we had just gotten back in time.

The saying *If you like something, why not do it twice,* is something that fits our girl scout troop perfectly. Each member of our troop was given the opportunity to plan a trip for the entire group. After sharing our trip ideas, we voted to see which one we wanted to go on. Abbey had planned a trip to Door County with kayaking, and hiking. I had never been to Door County so I was excited to go. Our only time to go was right before school started, our last adventure together before school. When we arrived, the place was older than expected and small but we made do and had the best time. We made dinner for our leaders and had a fire outside. The next day was a beautiful sunny day and the best weather for kayaking. We had tandem kayaks again and I was paired with Abbey.

The views we had while paddling in the clear water bay were amazing. We saw cliffs, rocks and had the opportunity to go into a small cave. It was cool.

When we passed the cliffs and saw a lot of people jumping into the water, we were told that after our experience we could drive or hike up to the top and go cliff jumping. I knew that was an opportunity I was going to hop on. We got back to land and decided that we would drive up to the location of where the cliff was to jump off.

Walking to the cliff and realizing how high up it was the nerves set in and I began to get nervous and unsure if I wanted to do it. The only thing that would ever set me back from something is the fear of something going wrong. When you look at the ledge from down in a kayak it doesn't look so bad but once you are up there looking down it can be pretty daunting. The whole troop told me that it would be fine, but Jordyn was the bravest and went first. Then I put my brave, adventure pants on and jumped in the water. We were told to jump feet first so that our hands, and arms didn't smack down on the water but as I entered the water my arms smacked the water really hard, and it hurt. I not only had the pain from smacking down, but I also had the realization of how cold the water actually was. When we were in the kayaks sweating it felt good but submerging our whole body in it made it freezing. I swam to the side and hung onto the rocks and watched everyone else in the troop go. It was really fun!

Once everyone was in the water, we all swam around to the other side where there was a whole "island" of rocks that you could sit or climb on to get back up to the top. We all did our own thing. Shortly before I decided to go again both Jordyn and Kendra had done their second jump. The only thing I didn't like about jumping more than once was how the water was so cold, and the fear of smacking my arms again but the jumping part was fun. I jumped and joined Jordyn and Kendra in the water under a tunnel cheering people. Person after person, some scared, some excited, some doing it for their first, some doing their third or fourth time, jumped into the water with us as their cheering section. After some time, I slowly started making my way back to the island of rocks and our leaders, Abbey and I started to climb back up to the top and were getting ready to leave and get food. Before we left, I had to jump a third time to feel satisfaction, while most of them said that they did it once and that was enough. They all thought I was crazy but knew that it was me and I was obviously crazy like that. As a reward for trying something out of most of our comfort zones we got ice cream. Later to wrap the night up we made dinner, a fire and played games.

The next day we had planned for us to go on a hike. We went on a short one that didn't take us that long, but we decided that we needed something more and that wasn't enough.

However, we didn't know what we were getting ourselves into when we started out on this hike. At first, we thought that the trail we were going on was just a short, easy, 2–3-mile hike all the way around. We four girls all looked at the map while our leaders checked in and agreed that the trail was going to be about 2 to 3 miles long total.

Shortly after we got started, we came upon a two-way path that was divided and we had to decide if we wanted to hike the difficult path or the normal path. We decided to go the difficult way because why not. We didn't know what difficult meant and so we wanted to see. Our leaders were not too sure about it but they left it up to us. Very quickly we were able to see what it meant. We went through some steep, narrow, and high places. We had to climb up and down spots and maneuver through rocks and cliffs. The trail ended up being longer and harder than we expected so it required a lot of grit, strength, and perseverance to get through the whole thing. All the tricky parts were hard for all of us, not just me. I could have given up but that is not who I was taught to be, so I kept moving. When it became difficult, we reminded each other why we were here and distracted ourselves by looking at the beautiful nature around us. To our left was the beautiful blue water we had kayaked on.

At one point we got off the trail and were walking on a main road and to change it up I would run down the road. I wanted to speed up our "2 mile" hike because I was tired and ready for the cool down swim. Before we made it back, we climbed up a couple flights of stairs to the top of a viewing platform and looked out at the beautiful blue waters.

"The best view comes after the hardest climb"

- Unknown

4 long, tough miles later we saw the beginning where we came in. We shared a treat, got our swimsuits on, and treated ourselves to a cold lake swim. The key to completing the hike was to keep moving and stay positive.

We also enjoyed escape rooms and TRYING to work together to figure out how to escape. Every trip, since our first time we tried to make it a priority to do an escape room because we have enjoyed them that much. On the trip we did one that was based off of the game Clue. We had to figure out who did it and in what room with what weapon. Just like the real game Clue there were different rooms with different clues, tasks, and hints that we had to figure out. We made it out, but barely.

To change up the fun our troop leaders planned a surprise trip for us. We had no idea what it was going to be about or what we were going to do, instead of telling us directly they created clues that we had to figure out. To also throw us off they gave us a packing list with some things that we didn't need. Personally, the only clue that I was able to figure out was that we were going to Chicago. On our way to Chicago, the leaders stopped at a house, and we had to put on some type of costume. We had no idea what type of costume, but we did have an area to pick from. As we were looking at all the options, we just picked out what we thought looked interesting/good on us and kept driving to Chicago. When we arrived in Chicago, we saw the Medieval Times Building and we knew that this was our destination. We were excited. In our costumes, we walked in and found our seats, and got a lot of compliments on our outfits. We ate dinner and watched the show from the front row with our VIP passes. It was amazing to watch the jousters riding horses, carrying swords and fighting. Some of the time there would only be two or three guys on a horse and some of the time there were 4 or 5 people going after each other. We watched white stallions that were trained to do trick routines and dance around in the arena. Even in our costumes we had a really fun trip and something I will always remember. Before heading home, we stopped and played some mini golf.

In appreciation, Abbey, Kendra, Jordyn and I always wanted to plan a trip that would surprise the leaders and with us all coming up on our last year in girl scouts this was the perfect time to do it, so we planned a trip to the Wisconsin Dells. Most of our trips have consisted of sleeping in tents, on the ground, on wooden slabs, etc.

so we made it a priority to stay in a nice Airbnb. However, that was our only plan that we had set in stone. We met together with Beth a few times to plan something but never left her house with any ideas in stone. The activities we thought of were just up in the air and we said that we were just going to wing it and go with how the weather was.

The day we left, on the way to the Airbnb, our leaders kept asking us what the plans were and where we were taking them and all we told them was that we would handle it and we had everything under control. They had no clue where we were going and even tried looking on google maps to see if they could spot any locations but were unsuccessful. A little less than 2 hours of driving later we told Jen, our leader, to turn onto this gravel road surrounded by trees and they were skeptical, but she kept going and pulled all the way to end of the road and parked in front of this small Airbnb that looked very nice and we got out and went to the door and they said "Is this where we are staying?" "Yes," we replied. They didn't believe us and when we got the door opened and stepped inside all of us including the leaders were in awe of how beautiful it was. We were proud because we did good. We were so used to sleeping in tents or on wooden slabs that it felt like a million dollars and the leaders thought we were fooling them, but we promised that we weren't. Once we toured our place and figured out sleeping arrangements, we made pizzas for dinner and enjoyed it at our nice long dining table together. After dinner we all played a board game called Pictureka for a couple hours and then our leaders went to their rooms to relax and go to bed, but we four girls had to have a conversation and discuss what our plans were going to be for the next day or two. We came up with the idea to go to Castle Rock beach for the day and spend lunch there and then go out to dinner that night at a nice restaurant and the following day on our way home we would do an escape room, but like our other trips the weather was not on our side. We woke up the next morning and it was raining outside, so we had to change our plans. Skeptical like the day before, while eating breakfast the leaders asked us what we had planned for the day, and we told them we didn't know quite yet because the weather ruined our original plans and we had to finalize them after breakfast. Instead of doing the escape room the next day we decided to do one or something similar that day. After searching and searching we saw Wizard Quest in the Dells and decided that we were going to do that. Wizard Quest is a place where you solve different clues and navigate to different rooms to solve these quests. Like an escape room but it has its own unique distinctions. Without the leaders still knowing what we were going to do we all hopped into the car and as soon as we tried to put navigation on, the speaker of the phone said, "En route to Wizard Quest." We all burst out laughing and the leaders knew what we were doing.

Once we arrived, we watched a quick tutorial video that explained our goal with the two hours of time that we had and we received our IPad. The IPad had different creatures that we needed to find/unlock. We got started and started navigating through a maze-like space with different rooms designed to the theme. For example, one room was water and so it was colored blue and had bubble lights, underwater creatures, and coral reefs and all the things that you could find in the water/ocean. In each of the rooms they had iPads on stands next to specific figures that had a story to go along. We watched the story and then answered a question that went along which then told us the next creature we had to find with the room it was in. It was fun and took a lot of back and forth and navigating but we did relatively well for some of us doing it for our first time. When the timer ran out, we went back and handed our tablets in and went to lunch. We chose Famous Dave's and wore amazing hats. After we were done and the rain stopped, we walked down the strip and decided to stop for ice cream at a candy shop on the way back to the car.

Back in the car, we drove to our Airbnb and rested for the rest of the afternoon. Some of us took a nap and others just layed and watched tv. We all just rested enough for the fun that came later that night. We blind folded the leaders and sat them outside on a chair and put a shower cap on their heads. It was funny. They had no idea what we were doing to them, and they were once again scared. After the shower caps were on we put whipped cream on their heads and started throwing cheeseballs trying to make it stick to the whipped cream. It got heated quickly and when the leaders figured out what it was it turned into a mini cheeseball fight between all 6 of us. To cap off the night, we tried to make a fire right after and due to the rain that day and the wood being outside we couldn't get the wood to burn and so we had to try and find dry sticks and newspaper to try to have a little fire. We were successful enough to make smores for us and then it started to sprinkle a little and we decided to go in and go to bed. The next day we headed home and ended our Wing It trip.

While it seems that all we do in girl scouts is fun and games (even though it is) we also have spent quite a bit of time over the years helping and serving others in our community. Every year for our cookie sales we chose a place that we wanted to donate our cookies to for our cookie share. We do the cookie share every year for people who like to support girl scouts but don't want to eat the cookies or can't eat the cookies for some reason. They can either donate money or buy cookies and donate them. At the end of the sale, we pick them out of our stack and deliver them to the group, business, or team we chose to donate them to. To name a few places that we have donated cookies in the past are the Beaver Dam Police/Fire Department, St. Vinny's in Beaver Dam, The Red Cross, Madison Children's Hospital, White Construction, Dodge County Humane Society, PAVE, chemo patients at the hospital and service men and women. Over the years we've been able to donate a large quantity of cookies. Seeing the joy that we brought to those people makes it a lot of fun and rewarding. Every single organization or group we have donated to has been grateful to receive them. The year that we decided to do the Red Cross we also helped and brought people food after they were done giving blood. It was a fun experience that we wanted to do again if the chance came, but we didn't.

Aside from donating Girl Scout cookies, we also made valentines for the grandmas and grandpas at the nursing home in Beaver Dam. One night we frosted cookies, and delivered the valentines to the residents, either in their room or in the main sitting area in the lobby. A lot of them told stories about what they used to do or what they were passionate about, their family. etc. I can't remember specific stories, but I do remember that Abbey went to deliver a cookie to a guy's room one time and was gone for a long time. As a troop we realized we hadn't seen her for a while and so when we walked into the room, we saw her sitting in a chair next to the man's bed talking to him. It was a special moment. Every year we were told that most of them really enjoyed having company in their room because they don't get that and so seeing someone and getting a special gift is so meaningful to them. They also loved the cookies. There were times when we were out at a table frosting cookies and some elderly people would come walking out and get so excited when they saw cookies being made. We left every time with a smile on our face feeling like we did something awesome.

Car care, coaching and another sports badge

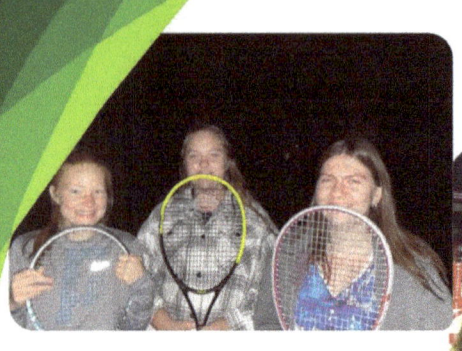

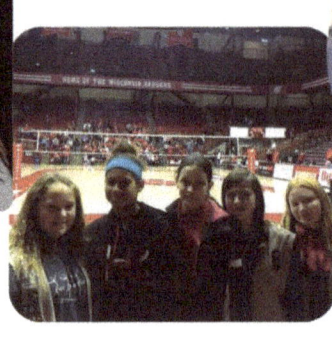

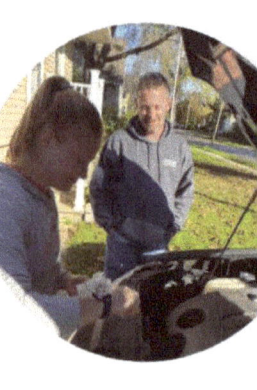

Tammy and I at one of our two cookie sale booths outside at Walmart.

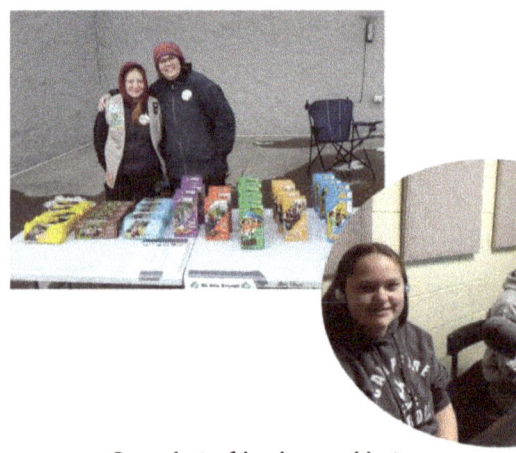

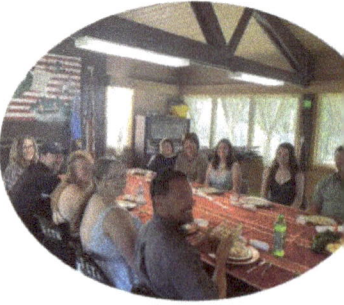

Our end of year dinner with our parents. We decided to wear ou prom dresses. Our whole meal was around foods we picked.

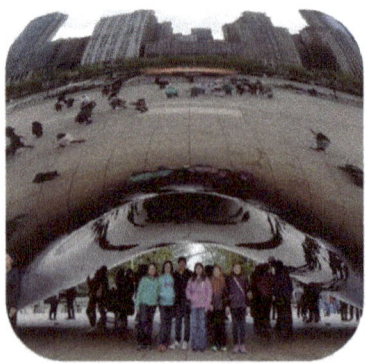

Snapshot of Jordyn and I at our radio broadcast to advertise our booth sale.

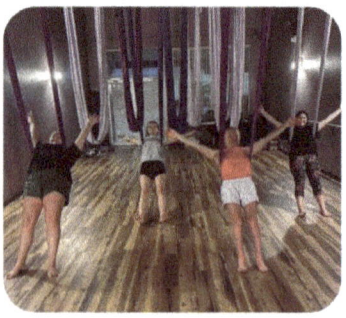

Some Yoga Fun for a girl scout meeting!

The Bean in Chicago. One of the big things that we made sure to see on our exploration around the city on our Girl Scout trip.

Girl Scout Week

Have you heard of Juliette Gordon Low? She was the founder of Girl Scouts, and every year Girl Scouts hosts a Girl Scout week where all the troops in Beaver Dam that want to participate in a window paint can. If a troop decides to paint a business's window, they first have to ask for permission to use the windows from the owners and then once given permission they have to decide what they want their "girl scout" window(s) to look like and create it. Then there are judges who go around and score all the windows based on certain categories and they announce the winner. As a troop we did that for many years. When we were younger, we had many more people, so we always asked businesses that had more windows but over the years we have gotten smaller and have not needed as many. Each year we've tried to do it around a certain theme that goes with that year and what we were doing. One year we did a horseback riding theme with a kayak, a girl scout sash with badges, a kayaker, and a music sheet with a girl scout song. Another year we did a "Shoot for the Cookies" theme and put hot air balloons, rockets, helicopters, etc. We did one with cookie wonder people with the theme as Wonder Women. Each year it became harder to come up with a design to do but we always figured something out. Our best year we created a tent and fire, with cookie people; some of the cookie people were ziplining and others were playing at a beach and kayaking. Topping the design off we put the phrase: Thanks-A-Lot 4 the Fun because that year was the last for the Thanks-A-Lot cookies. We loved our design, we thought for sure we would win it and it rained. The restaurant windows that we had painted were not covered by any awning or anything and the rain completely smeared and washed away our design the same night we made it. We were so upset because we knew that if the judges would have seen it, we would have won. Positively, one of the judges had driven by and noticed our window so we were at least able to get a rating from her and she loved the design, she thought it was very creative and cool.

Girl Scouts has truly been something in my life that I am grateful for. For all the experiences we have gotten to enjoy and go on is not something that I thought would happen. It has given me so many skills, lessons, friendships, and memories. Even though there are a lot more activities and trips that we have been able to do than listed, all of them are something that I will remember and be grateful for. Girl Scouts means fun, service, leadership, and growth.

Through my 13 years in girl scouts I can say that I have grown and loved every experience I have had with my former and current girls and my 2 leaders.

Family Cost: Priceless
The Ones Who Made It Possible

My parents had to find out the unfortunate news about my diagnosis and have little to no answers for most of the pregnancy. They had to expect the worst before they knew what I would exactly be like. During the pregnancy, my parents had the awful decision to either terminate the pregnancy or to keep the pregnancy going despite the circumstances that were up in the air at the time, but they always said that I was meant to be, and they would miscarry if I wasn't. They always believed in the process and knew I was coming for a reason. Always willing to do what it took to get me here safely and as healthy as possible. Once I arrived, they stayed with me and visited me until I was able to come home with them. My mom was unable to see me right away because of the c-section, but my dad stayed with me in the NICU, and my grandparents brought my brother in to visit. That evening, my mom was healed and rested and able to come see me again. The next day more family came and saw me. Relieved and happy that I arrived, my parents were ready to hear the prognosis and see what the next steps were in my journey. One of the very first things that I was associated with was many doctors from the UW hospital, who were there within a few short weeks I had been there. Once associated and hooked up with many doctors my parents went to appointments every few weeks and spent time talking to all of them that they needed to until they had some answers.

"Behind Every Young Child Who Believes in Herself Is a Parent Who Believed First."

Month after month, year after year, my parents lived with so many unknowns but knew the significance of my small accomplishments.

They never left anywhere thinking that they had all the answers. They were always looking for more ways to improve my abilities to be strong growing up and did anything that was required to keep me safe with no hesitation. The day that I learned to walk for the first time without a walker or any assistance, my parents were there to witness it and immediately called everyone else to let them know. All the independence that my parents taught me to have helped me be able to accomplish that small but huge goal and all the other milestones I have accomplished up until today.

While working, they have gone to sporting events of mine since I was little no matter what new one, I have wanted to try since starting high school. Even having a love/hate relationship with my powerlifting meets when they just have to sit there all-day and just cheer me on.

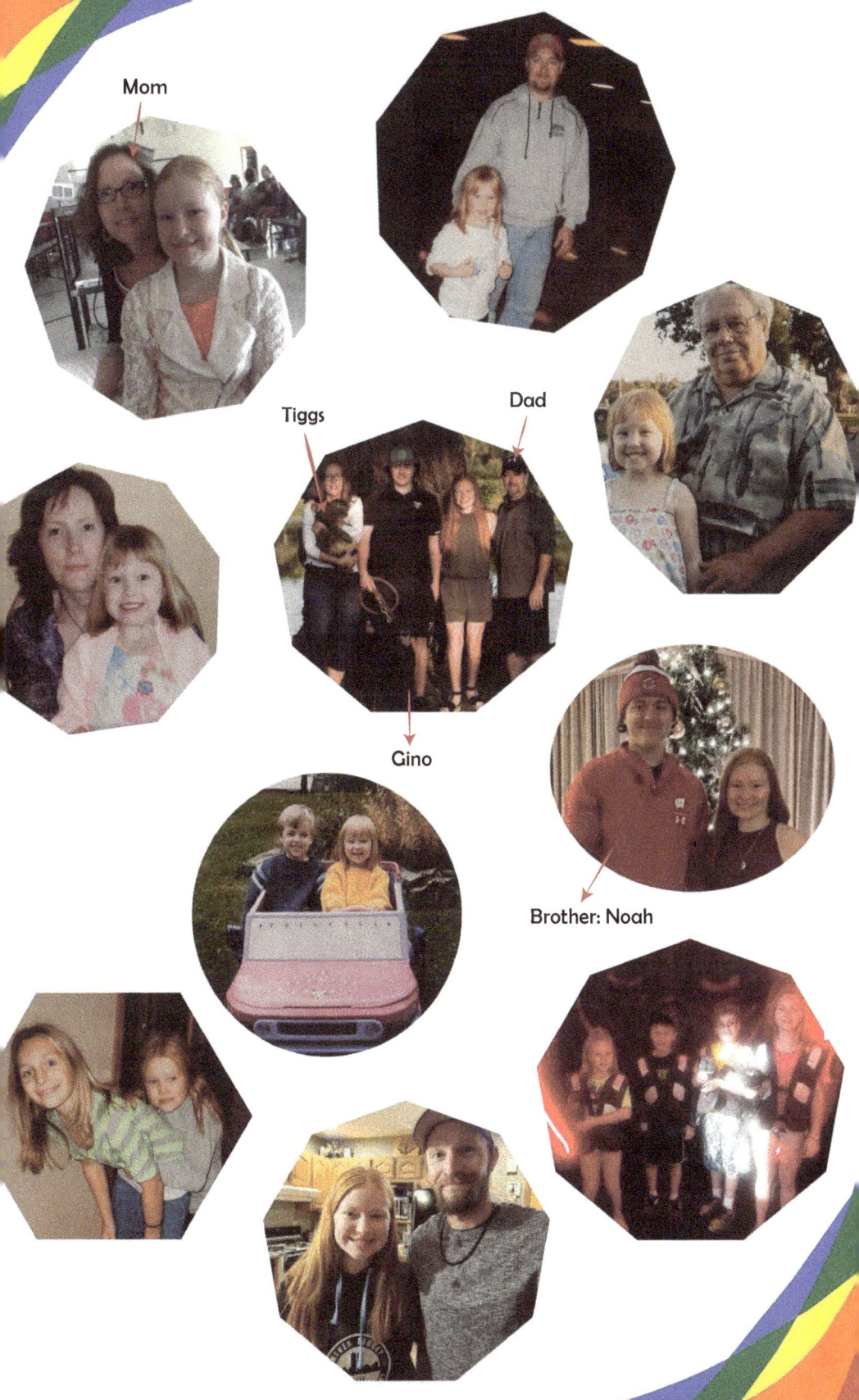

Mom

Dad

Tiggs

Gino

Brother: Noah

They've shown and told others that I can be myself and I don't need any extra assistance because they knew from the very beginning what I was capable of. If I got help, I wouldn't be the independent person they wanted and knew I could be. I have grown up to know how to have strength, confidence, drive, determination, and fight from them. They inspire me to keep going when things are tough. They had to mentally fight for about 6 months unsure of who their daughter was. Watching my parents strive for something they want and not give up is what makes me want to do things so that I can have the same opportunities that they give me. I learned from them that when I try something, I give my 100% and don't give up. They never expect me to be the best but the one having fun and giving my max effort because in their point of view just being able to do the things, they were told their daughter would most likely not be able to do is above and beyond.

They have provided us with so many opportunities including working at a very young age. When I was just 6 years old, I was able to start working at our family-owned campground, Willow Mill Campsite, in Rio, WI that was originally started in 1968 with my great-grandparents, which was taken over by my grandparents, and is now owned by my parents. Starting out I helped my grandma in the store stock the refrigerator and shelves, vacuum, check customers out, and put the ice cream away. At the time I loved what I was doing and looked forward to it every day. I was fine leaving all the dirtier work for the boys. As time went on and I became older, I started to transition to the stage where I wanted to do things that had me working both outside and inside such as hauling garbage, pulling weeds, reading meters, watering flowers, stocking the refrigerator, and cleaning the bathrooms. Currently to this day I work out outside mostly.

Every job has tasks that you don't enjoy doing but that are required. For me, that task is cleaning the bathrooms and watering the plants. These two jobs have never been my favorite because they are time consuming and not very fun to complete. I enjoy other tasks that take up more time than it does the bathrooms.

By doing outside jobs, I have been tasked with the responsibility to do more heavy-duty things including learning how to operate our lake weed cutter, to clean the lake for fishers, kayakers, canoers, paddle boaters, and a trimmer in order to be able to trim the grass.

Operating the weed cutter has been my favorite job to do ever since I learned how to operate it because it's easy, fun, relaxing and entertaining. For me seeing all the weeds that come up on the conveyor belt shows that I am doing it right and being efficient with my work and every once in a while I see a turtle, fish or both. I look forward to it every day when it's nice outside.

Just like at every job there is a routine every week of what needs to be done to clean up from the weekend and that includes picking up the garbage and cleaning the game room. Over the years my role with garbage pick up has changed and although every week may look different, I primarily help put bags back into the cans once the garbage has been taken out of it. Leaving the stinkier work for the boys or other girl workers. Once that job is done, we always spend the other half of the morning before lunch cleaning the game room. We have to vacuum the mini golf course, wipe down the counters/games, clean out any leftover popcorn that there might be, and sweep the floors. By then it is usually lunch time, and we take a break, eat lunch and usually split and do different things the rest of the afternoon.

The weekends are when the fun happens. I work hard during the week and then on the weekends I help and have fun. We always have a game room that is open on Friday and Saturday nights for the kids and adults who want to enjoy machine games, mini golf or free popcorn made by me (which people say mine is the best). It is always the place to be those two nights. I get to watch the little kids get so happy when they win a prize from one of the machines and sometimes both the kids and the parents get so into one of the games it is funny. There is one game called Drop the Hook where a couple families are very competitive, and they turn after turn try to get the shape in the hole and get so close but can't get it. It can be really funny and we can all get a good laugh, but some people are really good at it and others are unsuccessful. It makes for my long nights there that much more enjoyable.

The game room isn't the only fun we have for families on the weekends. We also have fun activities and events mostly every weekend. Some events that we traditionally have include a kids carnival, Rio EMS fundraiser, bingo, dances, trick or treating, etc. My favorite event, besides bingo, is the Rio EMS fundraiser. The day starts out with the EMS and Fire Department giving a demonstration of some of the things they do. Some years they have brought in their dive team and did a lifesaving/drowning demo, a house burning demo, CPR, etc. They serve brats/hot dogs/hamburgers with chips and cake while some of the camper's volunteer to sell raffle tickets, social basket tickets, and 50/50 tickets all day long. To wrap up the day we host an auction where people donate items and all the money raised throughout the entire day goes to them to improve their equipment or whatever they think needs improvement to make things more accessible for emergencies. Positively every year we have been able to increase the amount raised and the EMS and Fire Department are always grateful for what we do for them.

My last "job" on the weekends, if you want to call it that, is selling wood to the weekend campers. I load the wagon during the weekdays so that I can hook up the tractor and go right away on Friday night. When our campground is near full capacity on the weekends, I can usually sell a lot of wood and some weekends I need to reload in the same night.

Everything about it I enjoy doing. I enjoy driving, unloading the wood from the wagon, and taking it near their fire pit. It is one job that involves many parts of my body in order to get it done. It's like an easy, fun workout if you want to think of it that way. I love it and the campers are always so nice and helpful when it comes to unloading the wood.

Throughout all the different tasks that I have had to do I learned that I will need to use these tasks and strategies when I am older when I either go to college or after college and living on my own. Some may think that working at the campground is the only thing I am required to do because they only see me working there, it is not all that I do. Most days after work I have the opportunity to go swimming, kayaking, and hang with some of my friends and every weekend we host an event like bingo, kickball, or bean bags that I partake in. My parents are and have always been very appreciative of my work and reward me by letting me do other things away from the camp. I go by the motto work first, play and have fun later, but I love doing it and all the people I get to see and meet.

The independent, capable person I am is from growing up and learning from my parents what it's like to do things on your own and work hard. The opportunities in our lives that we have been given open many doors for the future for both my brother and I. Each and every day, both my parents tell me how proud they are of me and all that I do and lift my spirits in times where I feel low. We share many great stories about when I was younger and how scared they were of the unknown and what I was going to be like, but once seeing me knowing nothing was impossible. I know that they love to see me push past barriers that are bigger than me. I know how far I've come with them by my side and no matter what I do in my life they will continue to support me and be there if I need help or how far away I may be. They will always be one of my biggest supporting groups along with so many other family members.

I recognize every day how hard they work so that my life can not only be easier but also happier. All they have ever wanted is to provide my brother and I with a childhood/early adulthood that we will never forget. Something more than they were able to have when they were younger.

We have made memories on trips, through talks, and small experiences that show how committed they are to making our childhood that much more special. They've supported me in my newest journey as I make a big transition to college in the next year by giving me multiple options to choose from when it comes to deciding what college I want to attend.

I want them to know that there were and are going to be rough patches between us but every time we are able to push through and just focus on the good, the better and happier we'll be together. Our memories that we have created so far mean so much and something I will always have to look back on. They are the type of support that God knew I needed when I first came into this world.

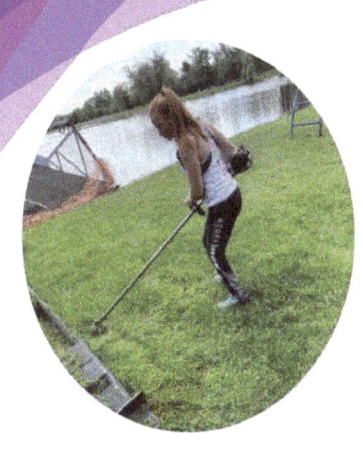

One of the few times I will ever trim the grass at the playground.

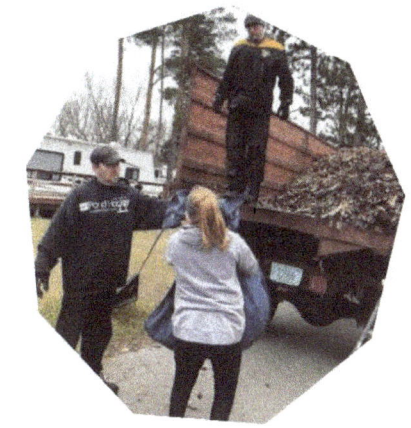

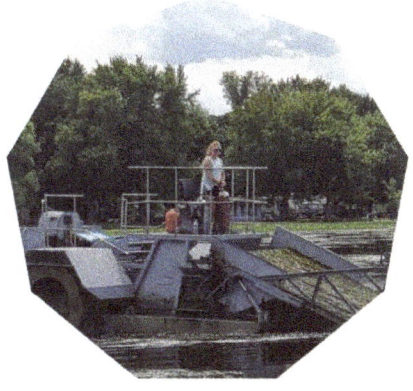

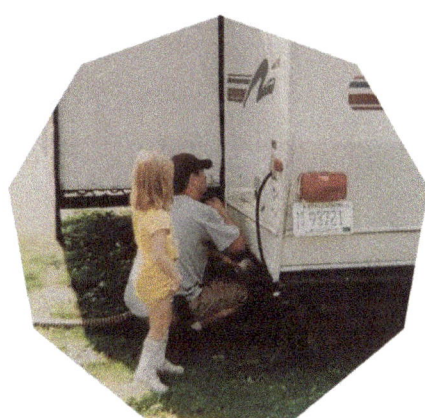

Future Pumper

One of the many times I operated the weed cutter in the lake.

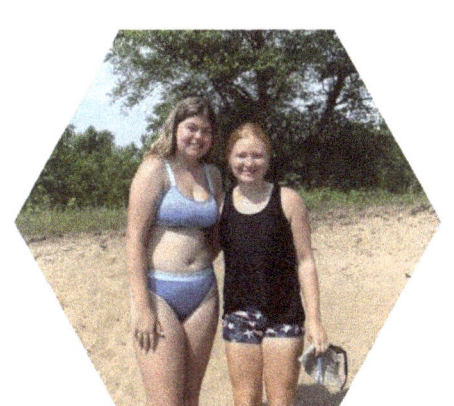

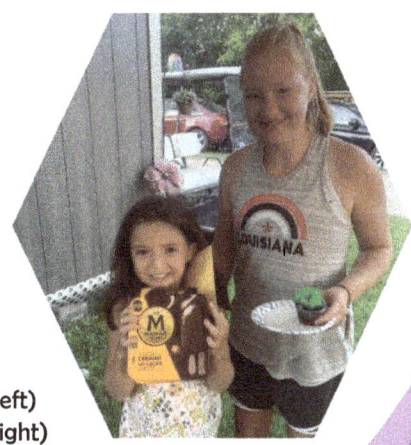

Cassie (left)
Addie (Right)

Camping Friends

Oh, Brother!

Siblings fight and siblings get along, and this repeats every day throughout their entire life, but what they have in common provides them with more good days than bad days. Same goes with me and my brother. We have gotten into a lot of arguments but since we have many things in common we are able to get along and motivate each other to be better than the other while having someone to rely on in any situation.

My brother, Noah, is two years older and for a few years we were in Day Care together. At that age being separated was so tough that whenever our class would go outside, I would go to the fence that separated our classes and stand there and cry because I wanted to be with him. The only thing he would be able to do was stand on the other side of the fence, close to me, because he felt bad. Eventually, he moved on and went to 4k, so we weren't together anymore, and I had to learn how to handle being alone. Thankfully I did.

Growing up, a lot of people said that I got my drive, determination, grit and motivation from always wanting to be better than or just as good as Noah. I agree. I never wanted him to win at anything we did together. Regularly we played mini hockey sticks on the floor or air hockey in our basement. Every time we did mini sticks, we set up the mini nets and sticks in our parent's room and played for at least an hour. Most of the time we got yelled at for being too loud or hitting the wall with the sticks, but it was so intense that it happened every time. It was very rare for one of us to come out of a game without a bruise or something hurting from poking and swinging the sticks trying to prevent a goal from going in. I would do anything to get a win against him even if it meant that I had to body check and shove him out of the way or flip my net over. Besides all the laughs we became more competitive and driven.

Mini Hockey became a popular activity that both my brother and I enjoyed but it wasn't the only thing that we did together to create fun. We played trivia, baseball, bowling, golf games on the Wii, hockey and golf on the PlayStation, and hockey on the Xbox. More games that would get pretty loud and crazy and my parents would be able to hear us. They said it sounded like an earthquake was upstairs because we would bang on the floor when something happened whether it be a goal let in by one of us or a good shot, homerun, etc., but it was just having fun together. Being in a love/hate relationship depending on who was winning.

Now with us being older we have gotten along much more and do things together a lot more. We have realized how much we have in common and used that pro to make it easier, and more fun to hangout, i.e., designing graphics on the computer, working out.

Since recently when I started getting into designing on the computer, he has helped me come up with ways that I can improve/enhance my designs to make it my best. He has given me techniques and tips that he has used before when creating his own work. The better the work comes out the happier I am because then I am able to not only create things for myself but also him and my parents.

When it comes to working out there is no bigger motivation and drive to do better than him than there is in anything else that we compete in. He unconsciously pushes me when I show up because the first thing I want to do is lift close, if not more weight than him. I work harder and have a stronger mentality than I probably ever would if I didn't have anyone else to go up against. He walks in with his best so the only thing that I can do to have the potential to go higher is to also bring my best and push myself to new heights. I realize that we are different, and our bodies handle things differently but that doesn't mean I can't and shouldn't push myself. He knows and I know that I can be strong and lift heavy. All the time we compare one another but we tell each other good job and laugh at our strengths and weaknesses. We have lifts that are definitely better than the other but that doesn't matter. We work on our own bodies and reach our own body's potential. He acknowledges if I tell him I did a certain weight but also assures me sometimes that I can do more weight. He says, "Come on Elizabeth, you can do more weight," and so the next round I try more weight and can usually do it and if not, I work up to it so that I can be able to in the near future.

Getting the opportunity to workout with him at the same time or on my own is awesome and something that I love to do because I know that there is no room to go less than 100%. I have gained a whole new perspective and a bigger determination and a "why am I there." Whether he's with me or not I am strong and can believe in myself and ask myself who am I getting stronger for, and the answer is always for myself. At the end of the day, it is for myself and with the support I am able to do that.

They say memories last a lifetime and the years go by fast and within the last couple of years it has really shown. We haven't been able to see each other as much so when we get the opportunity to do things just the two of us, we do, even if it is hockey related. He has always had the dream of playing in the NA3HL and that meant that he had to leave eventually. When his time came, we drove down as a family in his truck with all of his equipment and clothes and moved him into his place in Louisiana. It was cool to explore a new place but hard to leave.

The day before we left, just the two of us went and got food together and listened to our sibling song: Fight Night. We blasted it super loud and talked about work out and other fun memories that we have created over the years. We talked about him playing hockey and how he liked Louisiana. It was the best time we had together in a while and made leaving that much harder. It will be something I will never forget.

When Louisiana didn't fit, I went down with my mom and got him and headed to Decatur, Illinois, where he is currently continuing his hockey career. Having him closer to home has allowed us to have more days where we work out together, more car rides to hockey stores, more laughs, and memories.

"You don't get to choose your siblings. They are God's gift to you, as you are to them."

My Second Parents

I have been extremely fortunate to have a strong, good relationship with my aunt and uncle my whole life. They were just as worried, anxious, and nervous as my parents were when they got the news about their niece having Spina Bifida, but they were so excited to see me and to love me for the rest of my life. That was the beginning of our good relationship. Growing up they have treated me like their own and have come and see me do anything when they are available. They came and watched me swim at swim meets and my bridging ceremonies for girl scouts.

My uncle has had a job that gives him the opportunity to work in other states, but my aunt was always the one who took us to summer school. In the afternoons we would spend our time at her house and eat mac and cheese with hot dogs and play around. They have done so many things for not only me but my brother and cousins as well. They have and continue to help and be supportive. As you know most kids don't hang out with their parents very much, they prefer to hang out with friends or cousins. I enjoy hanging out with my aunt and uncle. I did when I was younger, and I enjoy it now. The times where my parents couldn't take me to a summer camp for something, my aunt would always be willing to take me and we wouldn't forget to stop and eat at Culver's and get ice cream. It was a blast. No matter how hard something may seem they always encourage me and push me to keep being more than I was the day before.

Some can say that I was like a magnet to my uncle when I was younger, but I love them both equally. Fun fact: we joke that they are my favorite aunt and uncle but realistically they are my only aunt and uncle but that doesn't take away from the fact that they are my favorite aunt and uncle because I am very blessed that I have them to look up to.

Anything new I have tried up until this point between swimming, soccer, and powerlifting and tennis, they were there both physically and in spirit. My junior year when I started playing tennis my aunt right away was willing to hit and play with me and give me more practice. Most days we were chasing after the ball in the next court, but it made for great laughs that were much needed. I have been very grateful that my aunt is willing to do anything with me whether I need a tennis partner, someone to cry to or just to talk and laugh with. She helped ease my mind by taking me to play tennis after the loss of my dog. She was there to make sure that I was ready for my first prom.

"An aunt & her niece… A bond that cannot be broken."

-Unknown

With my uncle working in other states our time seeing each other is limited and rare but the times we are together make up for it. Distance doesn't stop him from supporting, knowing, and encouraging me with the things I do. We communicate on the phone through Snapchat and hear stories of each other from the rest of the family. Holidays are when we get to spend the most time together. It makes the holidays that much more special for me and I love it. Every holiday I feel love from him, and I recognize the effort he puts in to seeing how I am and what I've been up to.

"The bond between an uncle and a niece knows no distance."

-Unknown

They both have always been in awe of the new things that I get to experience and encounter. They are proud and always bring positive words of encouragement. They love to see how much I do despite my limitations. They know that I take no shortcuts and strive to be my best.

All I Need Is Two

"Cousins are friends that will last forever."

-Constance Richards

Not everyone has a person in their family that experiences something traumatic or severe like a birth defect, accident, etc., so it can be hard for the family to live with that as the reality. When I was born, my cousin, Lauren, was two years old and my cousin, Michael, was only 3 months old so they were too young to understand entirely what their cousin had and how it was going to potentially affect their life. I grew up with their support and them being my friends. We always hung out together and had a lot of fun. They didn't have to include me in activities, but they always did without a second thought. During our elementary school years, we attended summer school together. Every morning they would make sure that I found my friends and waited for me at the end of the day, and then we went back to my aunt's house and hung out together. We rode bikes down to Waterworks Park and played on the playset, mini baseball, or on the tennis courts. The days we didn't play at the park we either went swimming or I hung out with Lauren in her room. No matter what, it was fun. I always knew I could rely on them if something happened and knew they would never exclude me.

As a tradition for Thanksgiving our family went to Kalahari for 3 nights or so. As soon as we got there, we wanted to go down to the waterpark. Lauren and I went off on our own and my brother and Michael went off on their own and all enjoyed the rides. She was always willing to go on any rides I wanted to and stuck with me and caught me when I fell. We always had fun. There would be multiple rides that we would continue to go on no matter what because of how fun they were.

They were busy as well and were not always available especially as we all got older, but they have been able to attend some of my soccer games and tennis matches to watch me and text me or see me on special occasions and check in on me if something is going on. They continue to support me and what I do no matter how extreme it may seem and are proud of all that I have accomplished. They are not only great cousins but also great role models for me and I look up to them in so many ways. The number of times we have laughed, played, talked, etc. are all memories that allow me to enjoy what life has given me and not even have a moment to think about what it could have been had my birth defect been worse. Not once have I wanted to change anything about my life, and I know it's because they have made an impact. They make family gatherings fun and are good sports when it comes to playing games at Christmas or Thanksgiving, especially when they don't know what they're doing. They truly have accepted me and done whatever it is to make me like any other family member. I wouldn't be the person I am today if they weren't so accepting and kind.

Cousins

Michael

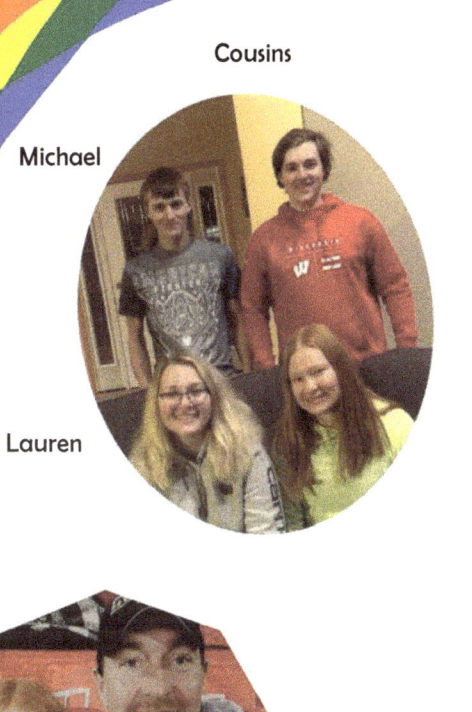

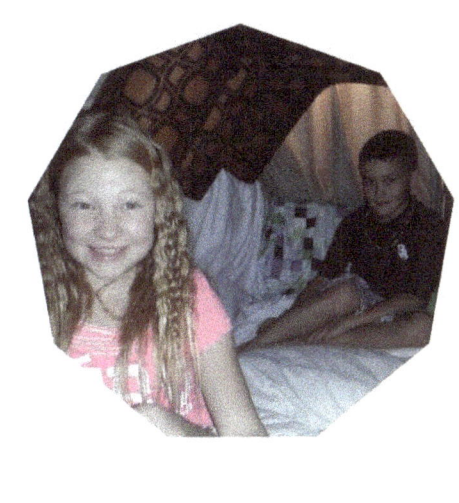

Lauren

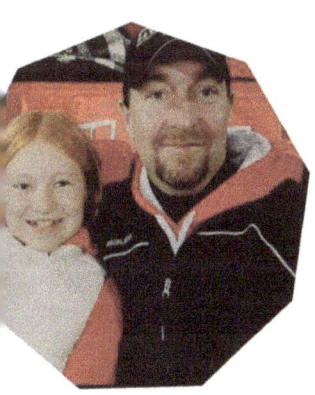

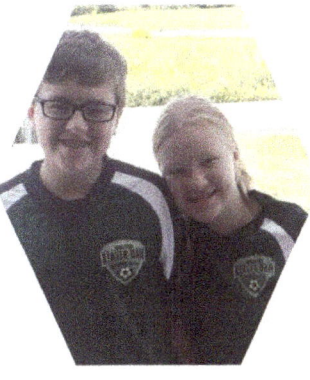

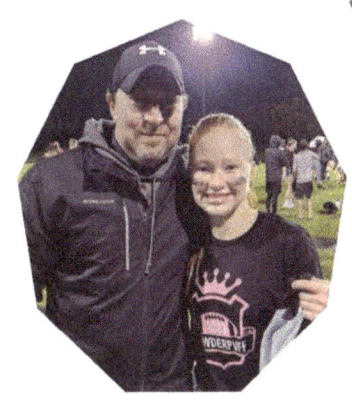

Grandparents (Dad's Side)

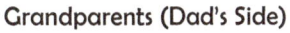

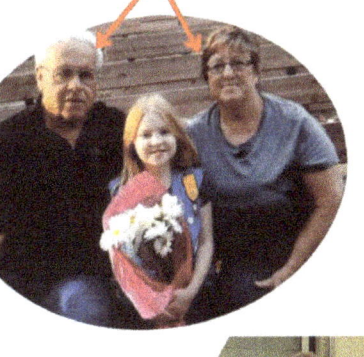

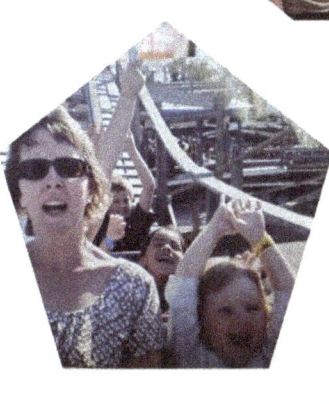

These Grandparents Are Fun

My dad's parents have been the grandparents that I have always had and grew up loving and knowing. Right from the start they were there for anything big or small. They have made time to come to my matches, games or meets to support me in what I want to do. Not once have they not been impressed, invested, and encouraging for all that I want to do and achieve. Every year that I have picked a new sport they wanted the schedule so they could come see me wherever it was, showing me that I made the right decision. I know not a day goes by that they are not in awe of what I have accomplished and continue to accomplish. They cannot believe what I am capable of doing. They never tell me or think that I can't do something, because they know that I will do it to prove people wrong. They show me how to grow up and support my family, welcome others, and have fun. I have learned and grown by watching them. They are the type of people who invite everyone in. They are the best hosts for all holidays and my grandma provides the most amazing food and treats for us to feast on. Every year for Easter her, my parents, aunt, uncle and grandpa would hide at least 40 eggs for all of us to find out in the yard. Even though most of the time we wouldn't find all of them we had a blast and loved it. She was also kind enough to make cookies for every holiday and send them to our class in elementary school and made sure there were extras for other teachers. The kids and teachers were always appreciative and always looked forward to "Grandma Banes'" cookies.

As I have gotten older and realized cooking and baking were becoming a passion of mine, I have been lucky enough to learn from her and have since made food for holidays.

For a couple of years now, my grandma has asked for help from my cousin Lauren and I to prepare Thanksgiving and Christmas dinner with her. We spend most of the day together learning and making delicious things. These learning memories make me have hope and excitement for the future that I will be able to create things just as good as she has. She has instilled a love for baking and cooking in me. No matter what I am doing she is always my loudest cheerleader on the sidelines and in the kitchen. She always has her camera in her hand so she doesn't miss any moment and can share it with us and others that love her. She even has a collection of "butt photos"." We joke every time she takes a picture that it will eventually go on the funeral board.

For all the moments I spend with my grandma baking, I spend my time with my grandpa in other places. He too just like my grandma loves watching all 4 of us grandkids playing a sport or doing an activity. He is invested in any match, meet or game I am in.

However, his natural habitat is working, and he works hard. When I was younger and he was the one driving the garbage truck, he would always ask me if I wanted to ride with him when he would go to the dump and unload it. Most of the time I said yes, and it would be a fun time. He would ask me if it smelled, and I always responded with yes. Once I learned how to drive the weed cutter, we occasionally would go out together and he would let me drive and he would just stand on the side and direct me if I got off the path. It was something that we both loved doing and were able to create memories from it.

Heading into college and getting acceptance letters has been exciting times for all of us. Each time I have shown them a new letter they get so excited and happy for me. They think that the process is a cool experience and I know that with whatever choice I have made they will come visit and support me whenever they can. Both my grandparents are willing to drive and do whatever they can to try and make time for each grandkid. They provide us with all we need and more. They make sure that we have everything and provide us with things even if we don't need it. Having grandparents that are willing to do anything to allow you to have an amazing life is something I won't take for granted. I enjoy spending time with them and sharing all my accomplishments with them. I know that without them I wouldn't be who I am and that they will support me no matter what life comes my way. Whatever path my life takes me I will think of them and have them in my back corner and use all the advice I learned from them to help me succeed. Especially when it comes to baking and working hard.

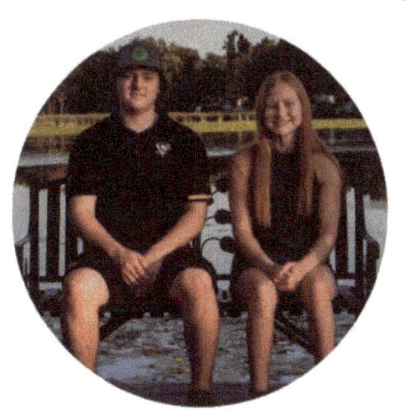

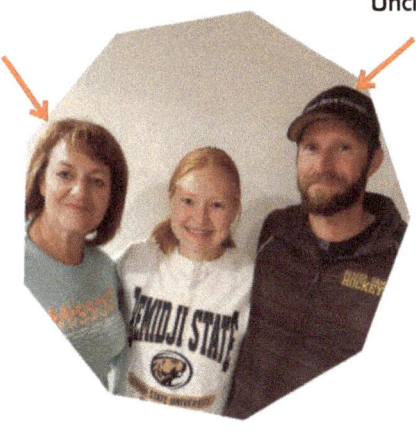

Aunt

Uncle

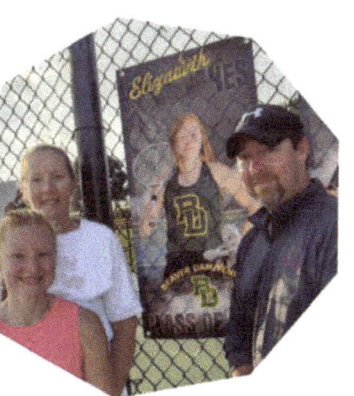

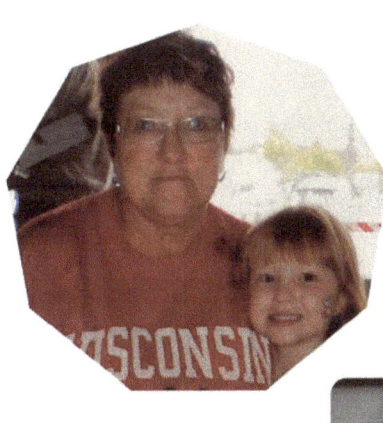

Aunt Barb

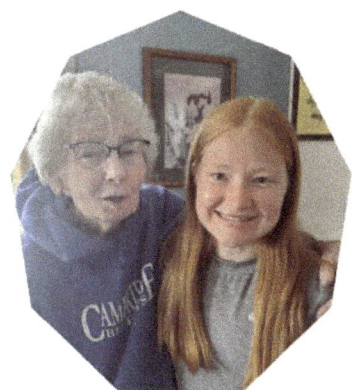

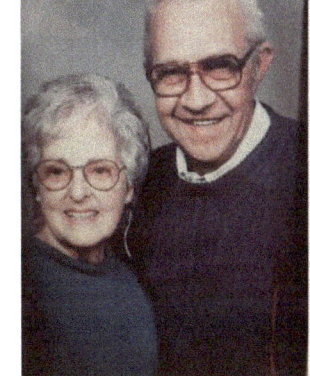

Grandparents (Mom's Side)

Uncle Buster

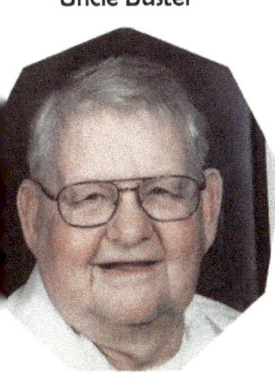

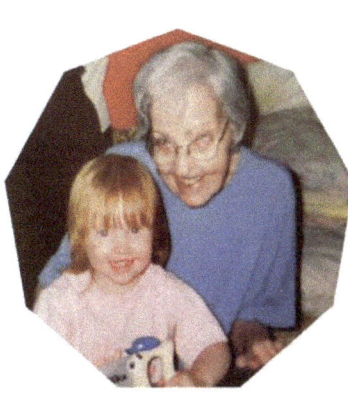

My Guardian Angels

"Grandparents are like stars. You don't always see them, but you know they're there."

-Unknown

Shortly before my mom found out she was having me her dad sadly passed away. Both my parents and the rest of my family were heartbroken with the news of his passing but with the exciting news about me they had a little joy. I believe I was sent down here by him so I could bring some comfort to everyone that loved and cared for him. I was the light to their dark time. For that reason, I was not fortunate to be able to know him but from the stories I hear I know that he was a great guy and was and would've been a wonderful grandpa to my brother and me. He cared for the people around him and did everything to make them better and happier. He loved hauling milk and even spent some of his life serving our country. He was and is a true hero.

To this day he is watching over me and proud of what I do. He is giving me the strength to be strong and have the perseverance that I wake up every day with. He knew that I would be able to handle a little adversity and knew nothing would stop me no matter how hard I would have to push. He may not be earthside he's living his next good life up in heaven.

On a happier note, my mom's mom was fortunate enough to live long enough to see me grow up until I was 5 years old. The day that I was released from the hospital we went straight to her house so she could meet her only granddaughter. We always visited with her a lot on the weekends and days where we were off school. She was older and wasn't able to move very well so I would sit at the table with her and talk. We played games, I showed her my work from daycare, colored with her, and just spent time making memories. She was proud of me then and I know she is proud of me now, watching us with my grandpa, cheering us on from the front row.

Two other angels of mine are my "other grandparents" on my mom's side that I was able to grow up with and I can recall more memories with. They are considered my great aunt and uncle, but they have treated me just like their own grandchild. They lived on a farm their whole life, loved everything farming and always had many animals.

My great uncle was a funny guy. He always made jokes and messed around with me at the table when we went to visit. Every time I would visit with him, he would have something to say or would try to get me to believe something I knew wasn't true. He always wore his overalls and snuck up on me like a spider. I loved every moment of it and never left without feeling happy.

When he passed away it was hard for his family and our family, but we honored him by visiting their house and his wife and sharing our memories and laughs just like before. His wife, my great aunt Barb, has always been an amazing woman. She has texted my mom, called my mom, and done everything to make sure that we get shown praise on special occasions. Every time we would visit, she would make sure that we didn't need anything or that she was up to date on all the new events in our lives. She would see Facebook posts my mom would do and get excited and be proud of us. She always showed she cared and made me feel loved. She was always in disbelief at me for what I was doing especially with lifting and now going for my Gold Award. Oh, my gold award. She loved that I was doing this book and talked about it every time I saw her and how much she wanted to read it and see it when I was done. Unfortunately, her health took a turn for the worse and unfortunately, she was unable to read it but the very last time that I was able to see her is a moment that I will never forget. She was alert and told me right away that she wasn't going to be able to read my book, so she said continue writing it and, in her honor, give it to one of her family members. I told her I would, and I would make her proud by writing it. Even with all that was going on, she still remembered that I was writing a book for girl scouts. It showed me that she truly cares for me and acknowledges what I am doing in my life and with that I know that I can do anything, and I will always have people supporting me like she did until the very end.

Adventures of a Lifetime

If there is one word to describe me and how I like to live my life I would say it would be **ADVENTUROUS**. Anyone who knows me knows that I love extreme activities and exploring new places and things. Spina Bifida hasn't stopped me from wanting to travel and explore and do some crazy things. My parents have blessed Noah and I and have taken us on multiple trips within the 18 and 20 years we have lived so far.

Disney

For Christmas one year our parents surprised Noah and I with mickey ears, which indicated that we were going to be going to Disney World. We were so excited and could not wait. It was our first time in Florida and for that our first time in Disney World. I personally didn't know what to expect and when we arrived it was nothing like I had ever thought of. I was young and all that came to my head when people would say Florida was beach and sand, so I thought that there was sand all over and no roads. I know, unrealistic, but again I was young and didn't know. We stayed on the Disney property at one of their hotels and was able to experience a lot of cool things. We went to all the parks, Animal Kingdom, Epcot, Magic Kingdom, and Hollywood Studios. I think that experiencing all the parks and rides, stores were super fun and amazing but going to Magic Kingdom and seeing the fireworks at night was the highlight of the trip for me. They had a new show every day and it was always themed and spectacular.

Washington D.C.

When my mom had family in Washington D.C., we were able to take a trip down there to not only visit them but also see the monuments, memorials, and museums. They took us around and showed us everything and gave us some history on it and what all the things we were seeing were. We were shown the space shuttle, the Arlington National Ceremony, the Abraham Lincoln Statue and the White House and the monument from the stairs. It was very sentimental to see all those important, historical pieces in person and know the history and stories behind it.

San Diego

In 2016 my family and I went on our first spring break trip out west to San Diego. I was so excited to go somewhere where it was warm, sunny and had a beach. We had planned something every day to explore and see. We stayed near the beach, so we had access to walk to it every day. Our first big place that we explored was Seaport Village. A little outdoor shopping place with seating, views of the water and a fire breather and sword swallower show. It was crazy. The most important part of Seaport Village is the USS Midway. The ship was located a little bit down on a boardwalk and you were able to go through all levels and learn about it. On the very top they had the planes and helicopters that were used and inside was all the pipes, concrete, etc. The whole village was super fun and loaded with people.

San Diego is also known to have a lot of seals, so much that they have a whole beach where it is just seals in La Jolla. The seals love it and just lay there all day.

After exploring the area around us for a couple days we decided to get more adventurous and go on something that we never did before. Dolphin and Whale Watching. On a small boat out in the ocean we went to look for whales and dolphins or any animal we could find. Our boat tour guide gave us information about what they usually see out on the waters and the history of the city around us. We started out slow and then increased faster and faster as we were on the hunt to find a spot where they were spotted. Unexpectedly we were able to find a pillar/buoy sticking out of the water with a whole bunch of seals laying out in the sun. For such a small area there were a lot of them. Shortly after we got super close to dolphins jumping in and out of the water. We all loved it.

What's a first-time trip to San Diego without going to the San Diego Zoo and SeaWorld? SeaWorld San Diego was full of amazing shows, animals, rides for everyone to enjoy. The show we watched was of orcas and dolphins doing flips and tricks. We lasted there for a couple of hours.

The zoo was no different. Just like SeaWorld they also had their specific animals in specified areas, just not polar bears, penguins, whales, etc. They had koalas, giraffes, elephants, tigers, etc. Since there were so many and the zoo was huge, we went on a tram tour to see them up close and even got the history and story behind them. Another cool way that we were able to experience them was by taking the cable car over the top of the whole zoo.

To end our last day, we went to the beach. I personally love hanging out at the beach on vacations instead of walking around different places, so it was nice to relax from a busy non-stop week. We had the entire day to go body surfing and play in the sand and jump into the waves. We had fun and I would've spent hours in the water if I could, but we had reservations for a sunset dinner cruise near our hotel. We had some delicious food, saw the most beautiful sunset, and spent time together right before we went home. It was a nice sendoff back home. This trip was where I realized my love for the beach and water sports was high.

San Diego

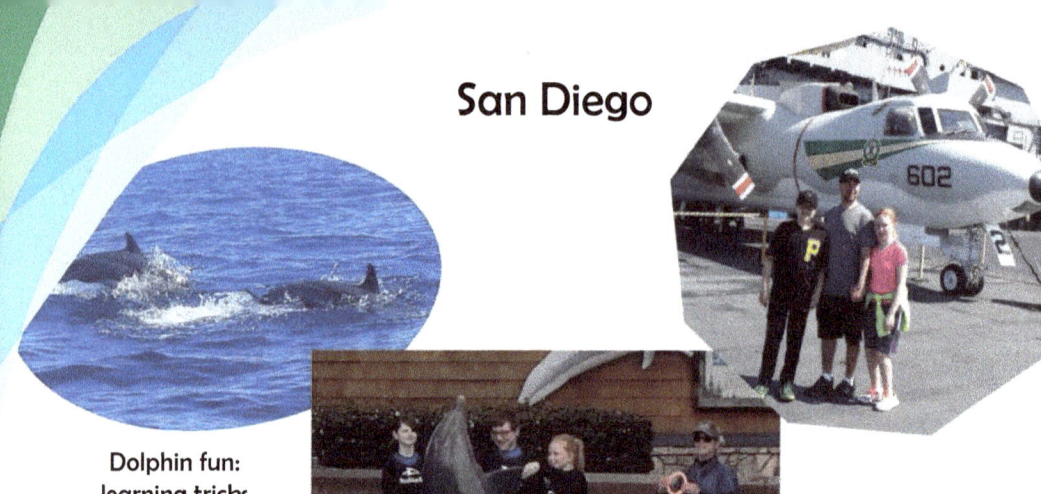

Dolphin fun: learning tricks and dolphin and whale watching boat ride.

USS Midway at Seaport Village.

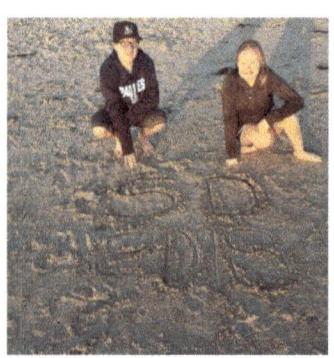

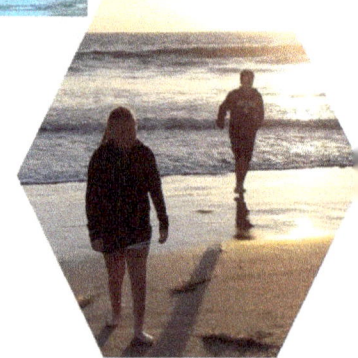

Beach Day!

Disney

Fun before going into the parks!

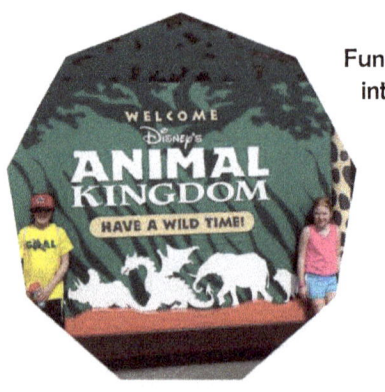

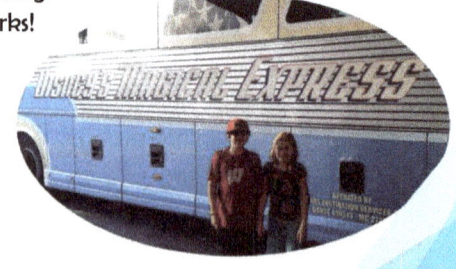

Myrtle Beach

A few years later after we tried out San Diego, we wanted a new place for Spring Break, so we chose Myrtle Beach. We had a few things that we knew we wanted to do again and try for the first time but otherwise we just wanted to take it one day at a time and figure when we were there what each day would hold. We wanted to keep it more chill and not so busy as before.

Most of our days we spent at the beach in the water, body surfing, jumping into the waves, or taking a walk on the boardwalk, but I did find places to go jet skiing, banana boating, gator sighting, and even found a place called Broadway by the Beach that had mini shops and restaurants.

This was the very first time that any of us had been on a jet ski and it was the best experience of my life. We had full range in a little canal to go wherever we wanted and do anything for an hour. They only limited how far down the canal we could go. At the time I was not old enough to drive so I was in the back of the jet ski and my dad was driving. My mom had her own and my brother had his own as well. From the very beginning I wanted to go faster but my dad was nervous that I would fall off or that we would tip so he said, "No, I am not going any faster." I tried everything but it didn't work. We stayed at the same pace, meanwhile my brother was long gone down the canal. The entire hour we kept riding and spinning and doing anything fun with them. When we got back, my brother and I said that we would absolutely do it again.

Fortunately, we rented Go Pros, so we have footage of us riding and later reviewed it. On the Go Pro that my dad and I used, all you heard was me yelling at him "go faster, go faster" and him replying "no, I don't want to make you fly off and I don't want to flip the jet ski over." Hysterically laughing already, when we got to my brothers, we heard him say "oh, look at that house" or "that's a nice golf course." It was a great time for all of us.

Our second first time experience that I wanted my family to go on was banana boating. We had no expectations but any that we could have had would have been wrong. Beforehand we were asked multiple times if we wanted to wear wetsuits and eventually my mom asked them if there was a reason why wetsuits would be necessary because we kept getting asked and the guy asked us where we were from and we mentioned Wisconsin and then he told us that we would be fine. The temp of the water would not have been anything different than we haven't experienced before.

Down by the dock, there was a boat that looked like a double banana with handles to hold on to and attached was a jet ski that would pull the boat around and make us go any direction that the jet ski went. Before loading onto the boat, we put goggles on, to prevent saltwater from getting in our eyes, and life jackets in case we lost grip or wanted to go into the water. Then individually my brother and I got on in the front and my parents behind us. After getting adjusted and ready, the guy on the jet ski started going and got faster and faster the farther out in the ocean we got. He made turns, twists, and all of us in the back were hanging on for dear life. We were laughing and having so much fun. There were a few turns that we thought one of us was going to fly out, but we all gripped the handles like our life was dependent on it. I wanted to keep going faster and faster, but my parents yelled no.

To give our arms a break he did stop in the middle of the ocean for a little bit, and we had the opportunity to go in the water then but no one else wanted to and I was unsure if I wanted to or not. It was an hour of fun that I wish to never forget.

When we got back to the dock the guy asked us if we had a great time and all we said was yes and we knew at that moment we would be doing another banana boat ride somewhere else.

After all the crazy, adventurous fun we decided that we would spend a day going to the Boardwalk by the Beach. A little place with rides, shops, and restaurants for families to enjoy. We walked around and went shopping and ended with dinner at a fun restaurant that was recommended to us by some friends: Dick's Last Resort. A restaurant that makes fun of you, and makes you wear paper hats with funny sayings on them. It's all supposed to be fun and jokes and not taken seriously. They have them all over and if you ever get the chance to go to one, I would recommend it.

Pittsburgh

My family is huge Pittsburgh hockey and football fans. When my parents met, my dad was a big fan and my mom watched the badgers and was a fan of the Czech Republic but that was it, so they began watching games together and even took multiple trips to go see them play in person. Then when both my brother and I were born they watched games with us and so we grew up loving them as well.

From a young age we have gone and seen the hockey team play both in Pittsburgh and other places and every time the experience just gets that much more cool, but our love for the city and going to Pittsburgh and watching them at PPG Paints Arena is so much higher. We have even been lucky to see a few baseball games.

Each of us have our favorite hockey players that we enjoy watching. Mine is Evgeni Malkin who I got the chance to get a photo taken with when I was younger, as well as a few other players. While most of our trips to Pittsburgh are to see games, there were also trips where we explored the city, toured different buildings and saw the Pirates play at PNC Park.

In 2016, this experience happened. The first thing we did when we got there was a duck tour (water boat that is like the Dells) through the city to learn the history and see bridges and buildings. The next day we were able to tour Heinz Field with a group of people and go inside the locker room, out by the field and even the press room area. It was very enjoyable and interesting to kind of see the life of a football player.

To bring our trip to an end we enjoyed a Padres vs Pirates game at PNC Park. We watched them during warmups get ready for the game and then we witnessed their team play together. It was a great game between both teams and made the night fun. After multiple trips to Pittsburgh after that I never thought I would go besides for hockey, but when the Wisconsin volleyball team made it to the Final Four and it was hosted in Pittsburgh, I knew I needed to go. I really loved watching them at the Fieldhouse and knew that I would love this experience in the city that we love most. My parents looked into it and my mom bought her and I a ticket for Pittsburgh for Christmas to go and watch them play. I was so excited to go I couldn't wait.

The day before their first game, the UW band had a pep rally outside at Market Square and all the fans that traveled were able to dance around and get excited for the days ahead. There were a lot of fans that traveled from Wisconsin to support the girls. After the pep rally we walked around the little shops and explored the city once more.

The next day we did some more sightseeing during the day and then went to a bigger pep rally at a bar, a block from PPG Paints Arena. It was packed with badger fans all decked out in badger gear, including us! There was literally no sitting or standing room except for on the stairs. It was crazy amazing the amount of support for the women. The coolest part I thought was that some of the parents and siblings of the players were at the bar and spoke to the fans thanking them for supporting their daughters. After some time, the UW band came through and played UW signature songs. It got even more electric and awesome.

When game time was upon, we walked over to the arena and waited until they opened the doors for us to go in. When the doors opened we walked to our seats and watched the team warm up and prepare for an amazing match. Their first game was against the number 1 ranked team Baylor. I knew that it would be a tough and evenly matched game, but it was nerve racking than anticipated. It went back and forth and each point was up in the air. The Badgers pulled through and won the match. We were so excited and ready for the championship game and see who they would go against. At the conclusion of the game, they made an announcement on the big screen that they would be signing autographs for a short period of time and so we jumped on it and made sure to get a spot in line. We waited and waited for the players to come out and eventually got to the beginning of the line where the players were seated at a table. They provided team posters to sign but I had a t-shirt that said *Point Wisconsin* on it and so I also got the players to sign that as well. When I got to my favorite players, I asked for a picture with them and got it. I thought standing right next to them was a dream come true. It made the night ten times better!

The day of the Championship was no different. We spent the day exploring and then got ready for the last and final pep rally at the bar again. It was just as packed and vibrant as the previous night. The difference was, after we spent time at the bar, everyone hurried over to the arena because they had a red carpet set up for the players to walk on as they headed in and prepared for the big match. Every fan lined up along the carpet and waited, if not an hour, 2 hours before, for the girls to pull up in the bus and come out and high five us. They always get escorted by police, with sirens blaring and lights flashing, so we were all listening and watching to see if we could hear or see any lights or sirens. At last, they came and everyone was ecstatic, had their phones out ready to record, and were screaming with joy. As the players got off the bus most gave high fives and little cheers of *let's go*! It was just as cool as them signing my shirt. Once the team was in the arena, we walked back to our seats that we had the previous night and waited for the game to start. This time they played Stanford. I knew that they would be good because they got to this point, but I thought since we beat the number 1 team, this team would be easier. Well, nope, not the case. It was intense and very unknown. Sadly, badgers couldn't stay with, and Stanford pulled through and beat them. It was tough and sad to see but they fought until the end and never gave up. I still thought that just having the experience of going to the game and seeing them play in the championship game was amazing. On our final day of being there we took the lift to the top of the city and got to overlook it at night and enjoyed ourselves some time at the little shops. It made me sad to leave but I knew I would be back again.

Pittsburgh

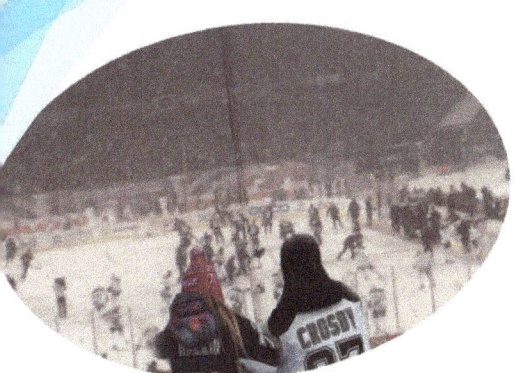

Outdoor hockey game in
a blizzard in Chicago.

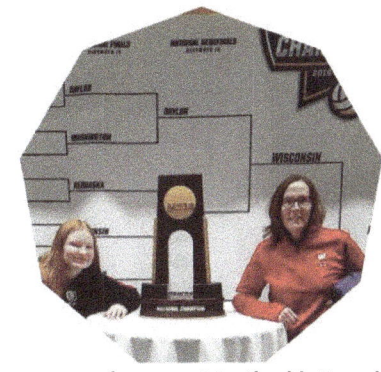

My mom and me next to the National
Champions trophy for college volleyball.

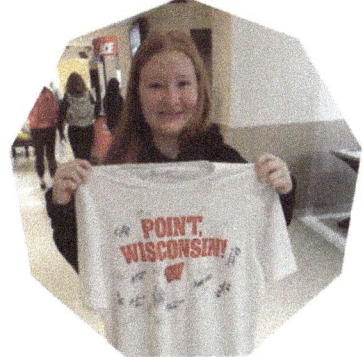

Holding a signed tshirt with all the
badger volleyball girls' signatures
after a meet and greet.

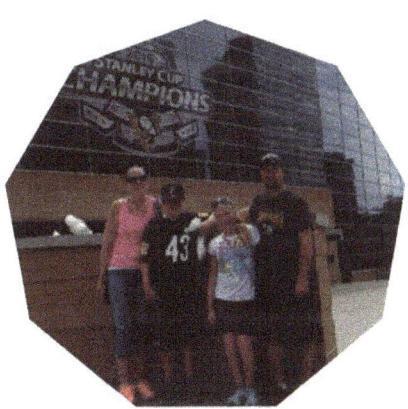

PPG Paints Arena

Alabama

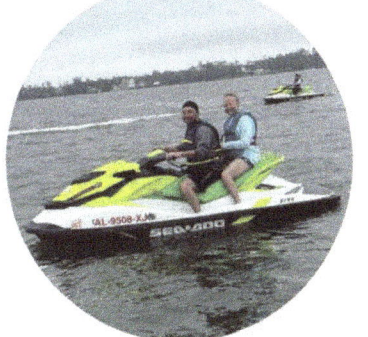

Jet skiing and beach
day with my parents.

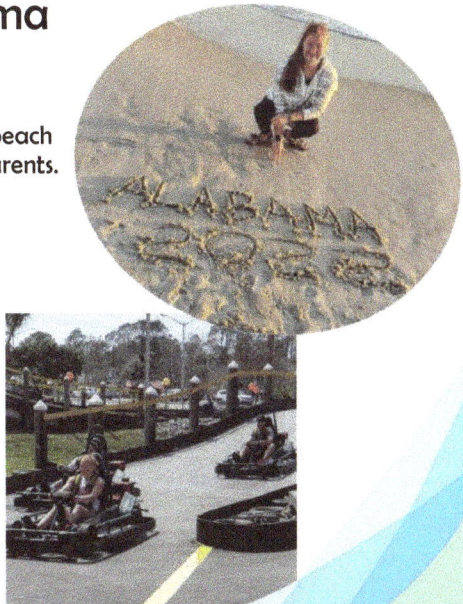

Axe
throwing
fun!

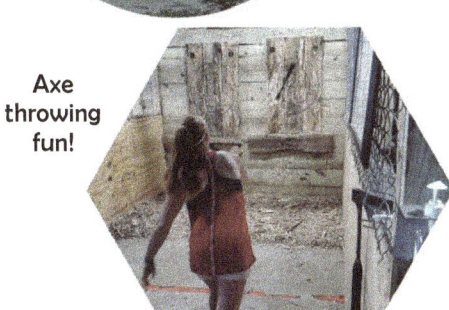

Philadelphia, Kansas City, Chicago

During the 2019 summer I started to really get invested in professional soccer. The National Women's Team was playing in the World Cup and ever since that tournament I have always watched them. The whole summer I planned my work around the games. If they played at 2:00, I was done working by 2 so I could watch the US play. I got really interested and loved it, most games I was on the edge of my seat cheering for them. I was just learning the players, but it was an experience I enjoyed watching. The first couple group stage games were a breeze for them but when they played Sweden, England, Spain, and the Netherlands in the final it was a battle. Despite that they won and held a celebration in New York. I was sad that I couldn't go to their celebration tour in New York, but I was hopeful that maybe I would be able to get to experience a game on their Victory Tour. Thankfully, right before school started again, they had a game scheduled in Philadelphia and my mom and dad were willing to buy tickets for me and my mom to see a game. I was so happy. We arrived there the day before the match and toured the city on the double decker bus and saw the banners they had hanging around town. The day of the game we spent the morning by the pool and then changed and got ready. I was so excited I had my World Cup Champions shirt on and counted down the minutes until the game. Inside the stadium they had merchandise shops that we looked at before we went to our seats to watch warm-ups.

As they were coming, I was in disbelief that I was looking at the women in person that I saw on tv not even a month before that. It was a realization that they were real human beings. Our seats were amazing and so was the whole game experience. They won and from that moment I wanted to go to another game.

The next time that I would be able to get that experience would be just recently for my 17th birthday. One of my all-time favorite players,

Carli Lloyd, was retiring from professional soccer and they were playing on a weekend that I had Friday off of school. I badly wanted to go and my parents were kind enough to drive me to Kansas City as a late birthday present. The 8-hour drive was definitely worth it.

We had a normal morning and then drove over to Children's Mercy Park, walked up to the stadium, and looked at new merchandise while we waited for us to be let in. About an hour before game time, they let us in and we went to our seats and took pictures of the field and of them warming up. This experience this time around was just as cool as the first and maybe even a little more because I knew all the players. Carli Lloyd did not start but she was subbed in around the 75th minute. The game ended in a 0-0 tie, but it was still enjoyable. At the conclusion of the game Carli Lloyd was doing her full field sprints to improve and get ready for the next game and it made me think of all that it takes to put in effort to improve and always wanting to be better. I had the thought that if I want to be just as good at something else, it will take more effort and discipline. It was super cool to see her do that.

Leaving the game in Kansas City I thought that it would be the last time to see Carli Lloyd play but it wasn't. She and most of the other girls are also a part of a club team in the National Women's Soccer League. She played for Gotham FC in her hometown New York/New Jersey. They made it to the playoffs and their first game was against the Chicago Red Stars with the Red Stars hosting it. As soon as I saw that, I said, "Mom, they're playing in Chicago. The tickets aren't that much. The drive to Chicago isn't that far. Can we please go and see them play in Chicago? I promise this will be the last time we go see soccer in person for a while." After a little convincing they agreed, and we bought our tickets to the Red Stars vs. Gotham FC game. I was so ready that I made her a sign that I was hoping to get signed.

We drove up on a beautiful sunny day and got there in time to watch warm-ups. As soon as we sat down, I looked at my mom and was in awe. We were in the front row in the corner of the stadium. I couldn't believe that we got so close to the field. After warm-ups were done the game started and it was evenly matched throughout. Each team had their chances but couldn't finish any of them. I really liked both teams, but I was rooting for Carli. My favorite goalkeeper and player on the Red Stars weren't playing so I wanted Gotham to win. At half time they were tied 0-0 so we knew that it would come down to the very end to see who would advance. With only about 20 minutes to go, Chicago was able to take control of the ball and Mallory Pugh, one of the national team players, dribbled the ball down the field and shot and ended up scoring. It was now 1-0 Red Stars and all I wanted so badly was for Carli to get a goal and tie the game. She had opportunities but could never capitalize on them enough to score.

You could see in her face that she knew the clock was ticking down. They lost and that was her official final game in any soccer uniform.

Following the game, they had autograph signings for the fans. Some of the players walked around and signed jerseys, pamphlets, anything that you had. Since we were on the Chicago side most of the players from the Red Stars were signing our items. I was hoping to see Carli Lloyd and get her to sign my poster and jersey, but she never came on our side and eventually it was too late, she went back to the locker room. However, on our way out I saw these two people and I said to my mom "Hey, that's Carli Lloyd's parents over there." She replied with "Where, go up to them," but I was too shy and told her to and so she sped up a little bit and we met them right by the top of the steps. She asked them if they were Carli's parents and they replied with yes. So, we walked down the stairs and talked to her parents for a little bit and I was able to show them my sign that I made for her and they took a picture of me with it and said that they would show Carli. They were so nice, and I ended my trip extremely happy.

Philadelphia, Kansas City, &
Chicago Soccer games

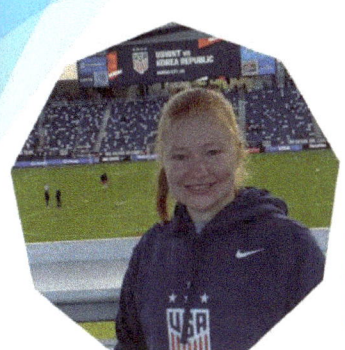

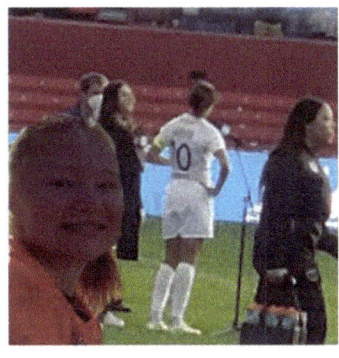

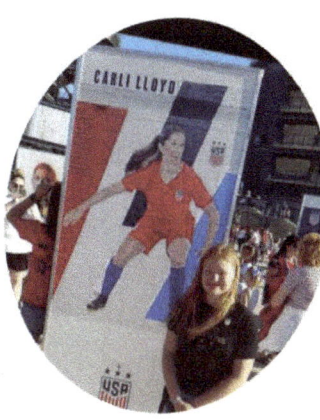

Myrtle Beach: Parasailing
with my family, beach days
(body surfing)

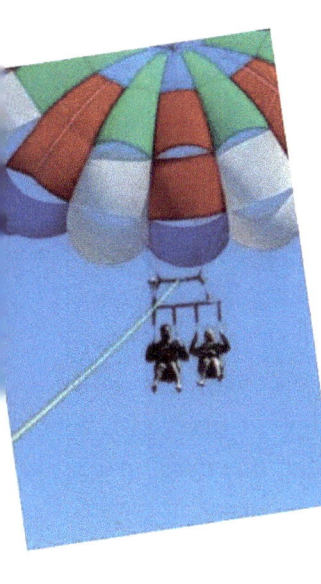

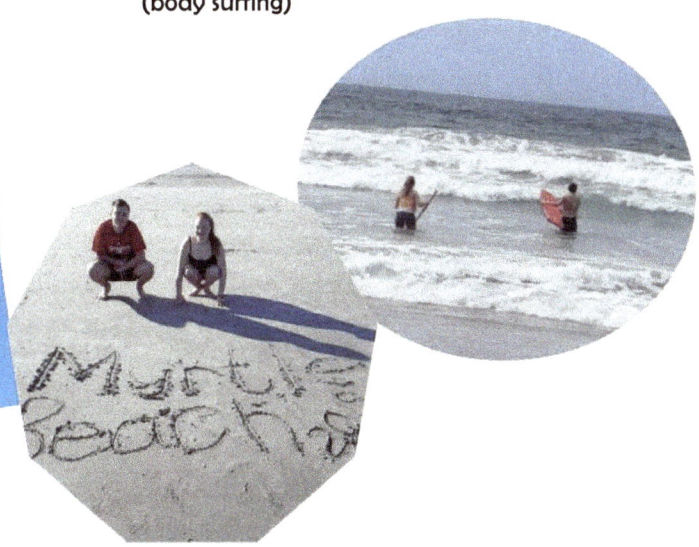

Alabama

All our spring break trips have been with all four of us together. This time my brother had just wrapped up his hockey season and didn't want to go so I was able to choose where to go. I chose Alabama. It looked very warm, sunny and the beaches looked white. Flights were astronomical so we drove. We took our beach chairs, towels, anything essential that we needed. On the drive down we stopped to sleep once for a couple hours but then kept going. Every state we went through it was cool to see the skyscrapers, and scenery around us. The drive was long, but it was beautiful.

The trip was called the Three Musketeer trip because it was only my parents and I (everything we did was a three musketeers experience). We arrived in the late afternoon and took a stroll down to the beach to step our feet into the water and got rested for the adventures for the week. Before we got into anything crazy and adventurous, we drove down to The Wharf and walked around and in and out of shops. We saw what it had to offer and saw that it had activities we wanted to do later in our trip. The first big adventure that I planned was jet skiing out on the ocean to find whales and dolphins. The morning was cold and overcast which made it difficult to get the dolphins and whales to wake up so we could see them, but I didn't mind that we just rode around. We took quite a bit of time to try and locate dolphins or whales but again the weather was just not on our side. After casually cruising at a normal speed, we got to an area where our guide allowed us to roam free for a little bit and do anything and everything we wanted. My dad and I, on our jet ski, went in circles, and did twists and turns. It was what I wanted to experience. It made up for not seeing any dolphins.

Quickly after we had to head over to a beach where they were offering banana boating. On our way the weather started to clear up and the sun came out making it warmer outside. The hopes of having good weather for banana boating increased drastically.

If you compare this banana boat ride to the very first time we did it, it was very different. The "boat" was an inflatable raft and inside was the banana shaped floatie with handles. It was safer and more protective than the other. It was interesting to get on because the water was so wavy, and as you were trying to get on the waves would push us and the raft away from each other.

We made it on successfully and started going right away. The whole time we were laughing and having fun but by the end our arms were sore from holding on. I would have kept going if it was up to me but everyone else was ready to be done.

To keep our trip relaxing we tried to spend at least a little time at the beach each day whether it was in the more or after excursions, but some days were more of a challenge when the wind was strong creating a chillier breeze. One day the wind was so bad that our water activities were postponed, so we redirected our fun somewhere else. We found Adventure Island and spent the day go karting, mini golfing, playing arcade games, and driving bumper boats. My dad and I did go karting and I was leading until one of the last couple laps when I was taken out by someone else and then got stuck in the corner and turned sideways. Our favorite: the bumper boats, were a blast. We had other people with us who were just as invested in spraying others as we were. It seemed like everyone was targeting me with their water which was unfair, but it was fun.

The end of our trip was rainy, so we planned to do our ax throwing and escape room. It was my dad's first time in an escape room, but my mom had done one before and I had done several so I felt confident that we could escape. Our theme was a deserted island and we had to try to escape before a volcano erupted. We did decent for not doing one together before, but we were not able to escape.

Ax throwing none of us had done before and so we took a few practice tries before trying to do a competition. We weren't terrible at it but also not pros. I either stuck it or it would hit it and bounce off. After a little time, I decided to start the competition and keep track of our points. My dad did the best but as we progressed all of us were able to nail it especially in the higher points region. We laughed and laughed and had fun for 2 hours while it was raining outside.

Every trip we like to end with something new/fun. We decided to do a glass bottom kayak sunset tour. We were supposed to set out at sunset and go paddle around on the water and find some sea life, but it only ended up being a short 8–10-minute kayak tour looking for snails on a little island. I didn't find anything, but I think some people in our group found some snails.

New York City

Every year on New Year's Eve, either in person or on TV, everyone stays up until midnight and watches the ball drop at Times Square in New York City. Recently I was able to see the ball thanks to my grandma. She has always wanted to go and with all of us hitting big milestones this past year she gifted my aunt, cousin, mom, and I with a trip to New York. As the days were approaching, I was super excited and knew that it would be fun traveling with them, but I didn't know it was going to be as fun as it was.

Our very first day started out with a crazy, adventure filled ride to our hotel in downtown Manhattan. After arriving at our hotel, we had lunch, rested, and set out to explore New York for the night. The first place we walked to was Rockefeller Plaza to see the Christmas Tree, the ice rink, and a light show on the building next to the Cathedral. It was crazy busy and full of people exploring and having fun.

Inside the plaza they have shops, and restaurants you can eat at and windows to view the ice rink. We loved it and thought that it was the most beautiful thing we ever saw. On our way back to the hotel we passed shops and places we planned to stop at later on in our trip.

The next day, the first official day, was the day that all the big events and sightseeing tours began. We started out early, went to breakfast next door, and walked to find the subway. We had a few times where we went the wrong way and even happened to walk up to Times Square and see the Good Morning America building and the 2022 ball but we found the subway and got on. It was our first experience with the Subway so we were cautious to make sure we got off at the right stop. We got off and were only 3 blocks from the 9-11 Memorial, so we did well. We decided to tour the memorial independently which allowed us to read the stories and look at the artifacts at our own pace. The first display was a picture of the city the morning of the attack and on the wall across from that was the routes of the flights that were a part of what happened that morning.

As we continued, we saw pieces of steel and concrete from the Twin Towers that were destroyed. The whole place was silent as people reflected on that day and what they were able to salvage. These beautiful things were created from an event that was so terrible and horrifying to millions of people. They really had so many pieces and creative ways that they were able to honor not only those two buildings but also the people and the families of those people that lost their lives that day.

One of my favorite walls read,

"No day shall erase you from the memory of time"

-Virgil

The words are made of steel salvaged from the wreckage and around the letters are watercolor square tiles with all shades of blue with the remains of the ones who perished. It was neat.

Next to the wall is a room filled with 4 walls covered in tiles with pictures of those same people and their names and displays of pictures and artifacts that the family kept and displayed for the world to see. They represent what their favorite things used to be. As I was walking through it was just so amazing to see things so beautifully thought out for these people and their families.

The theme of the whole exhibit was damaged, dented, reused. It was crazy how things looked. Some were hardly recognizable like the very first fire truck that was on scene that day. I could not help but think how frightening it would have been to be a firefighter/dog/human near it that day. Everyone was a hero and gave their life that day.

My favorite part of the memorial was the display section of all the 9/11 therapy, service, and recovery dogs. I am a dog lover, so this section made me emotional. There were a lot of dogs that played different roles in helping bystanders, firefighters, and anyone they could. It was sentimental and a place where I knew the real role of dogs and why they are so comforting and loving. No matter what situation they were put in, they did their job and did it well.

"Those who teach the most about humanity aren't always human."

-Donald L. Hicks

After the memorial, before walking back to the Top of the Rock Observatory at Rockefeller Plaza, we quickly stopped at Carlo's Bake Shop, and each picked out a dessert. Why dessert? Well, what is being adventurous without a little treat to go along with all the fun and who doesn't want to say that they have eaten something from Buddy's (Cake Boss) shop. Not me. After a lot of choices, I chose to get a brownie and share it with my mom. It was delicious. Once we returned to Rockefeller Plaza, it was time for the Top of the Rock Observatory. The Top of the Rock did not disappoint. We started out by taking the elevators to nearly the top floor. When the elevator doors opened and we stepped out, all around us were glass windows with miles and miles of the city of New York. I remained fearless and we went outside and saw NYC from a different perspective.

Every day from the day we got there and the day we left we were finding new ways and shorter paths to get everywhere. As we were looking out, we realized that we could see the ball in Times Square and laughed because we didn't realize we were so close. With more height to explore, we took the escalators to the top floor and walked out and around the whole thing at the highest point possible to view the city. I found it so fascinating to see all the tall buildings and billboards from so high up and I loved how far out and how much of New York you could see.

On our way back we stopped at Rockefeller Plaza to see the NBC store, Jimmy Fallon's Door and to have lunch and ice cream. After running into Time Square by accident while trying to find the subway, we made it a priority to come back that night. There were many different stores, shops, and outlets for everyone. We went there to not only see the ball but to go to the Hershey's Chocolate Store. Just walking in there was mind blowing and cool. We were greeted with mini Hershey bars and surrounded by many humongous sized candy bars. Every type of candy/candy bar that you could possibly think of was in the store in giant size. There were Hershey bar flavors in there that I never had even heard of that sounded really good. My cousin and I were upset that we had ice cream earlier because they had a mini ice cream shop in the store and a s'mores station with the chocolate being different bar flavors. From the pictures it looked amazing, but we didn't try it out. Instead, we bought candy to bring back to the hotel to try.

Our candy loving sensation wasn't quite calmed yet and right across the street was a bright m&m sign calling our name, so we also stopped. It was massive with 3 stories and every wall lined with either m&m clothes or tubes filled with different colors and flavored m&m's that you purchase in a bag. They had tons and tons of flavors/colors, about 30 on each level. The place was packed with children and parents loading bags and bags full of m&m' s.

Since Time Square is the place to be, there were small huts/shops with all kinds of accessories that you could think of. Everywhere I go I get two things for sure, a snow globe and something from Hard Rock Cafe. I found one I liked and bought it as a great memory.

Shortly down from them was Hard Rock Cafe. I usually get a sweatshirt but as I was looking, I found something even cooler. A t-shirt of Times Square all lit up with bright colors, billboards, and the ball. Once we were all ready to be done shopping around at Times Square, we went to a late dinner at Smashburger and went back to our hotel.

Day 3 of our trip had only one scheduled event: Empire State Building! We were tired from going, going, going the day before so we were happy, we only had one thing and then were on our own to make plans. Walking through the ground level they had mini replicas of the Empire State Building and videos of the process of building the structure. Near the elevators they had a structure with King Kong's fingers sticking out of the building where my cousin and I got a picture taken.

We got to the first set of elevators that took us to floor 80 but we wanted the view from the outside, so we took the escalators up another 6 levels. The views were all the way around and gorgeous. We again saw miles and miles of the city, The Edge, Madison Square Garden and the world's largest store, Macy's, which we visited next.

The store has about 8 levels with a whole range of shops for all ages. Most of it is too expensive for us Wisconsin people.

As exhausted as we were from going long the two nights before and walking all day long, we made a trip back to the hotel to rest for a couple hours before my aunt, cousin, mom, and I went back out for the night. There were places that they wanted to see and so we decided to go out and have some more fun. Our first place we headed to was FAO Schwarz; the toy store in the movie Big. Trying to get there was like a lost person trying to navigate through a maze. There were even more people it seemed out that night and trying to move in any direction was hard. After kindly pushing and navigating through, I got us to the store. They had multiple stories of toys, stuffed animals, dolls, etc. all over for little kids. On the top story, there was a floor piano with kids playing on it. Out of the store, we headed to dinner where it was more nonstop laughing.

You would think after that we would be done with walking, especially after walking about 20,000 steps a day but no, we wanted to see Madison Square Garden since we saw it from the Empire State Building. It was about a 12-minute walk, but we didn't care. When we got there, and the store and doors were locked and officers were guarding them but we caught a glimpse of an ornament hanging from the roof of the New York Rangers logo.

Our last full day in NYC began with a cruise to the Statue of Liberty. The morning started out rocky, but we got there with 5 minutes to spare. Right from the beginning I loved it. I love boat rides and anything with water but the most amazing part for me was when I was standing outside in the front of the boat. It was cold but when I love something I just don't care. I just stood out there and looked around. Meanwhile our captain talked about the history of the buildings and the different things around us.

As we were approaching the Statue of Liberty more people came, including the rest of my family. We took pictures and took it in because it was right in front of us. Most people know what it looks like from pictures and tv, etc. but to be able to see it in person for me personally was super cool.

Central Park was the next thing that my aunt, grandma and mom wanted to see so we caught the subway again and went to Central Park. We entered and just started walking. We were told that it was 6 miles all the way around, but it didn't faze us. We weren't too far in when we stopped to take pictures and I was given a map that helped guide us through the park. It may have been a little bit confusing at first, but I figured it out and got us going right. Walking all 6 of those miles was too much for all of us but the trees and scenery we saw on the walk were beautiful and worth every step, pain, soreness, etc. It was still overcast so it was just the right temperature out. Every now and then it was sprinkling but for the most part it was cloudy. After walking all our snacks off we were hungry and tired. We got back to the subway and sat down and oh did it feel good. Back at our location we grabbed a bite to eat near our hotel and ended with tons of laughs and funny stories.

The morning of our departure my mom and I went to breakfast at a diner that we went to the night before and then got back and packed up our stuff. Then we did some shopping around our hotel before it came close to the time our ride was picking us up. We were scheduled to get picked up at 2. However, the vehicle that came and picked us up had a misconception and thought that we only had 3 people, but we had 5 and a lot of luggage so there wasn't enough room. They ended up not having any more vehicles available to get us to the airport, so a cab was called and caused another problem. The cab was pretty much the same size as the car that had originally wanted to pick us up, but after a little convincing we were able to get the driver to allow us to all fit in and take us to the airport. It was a little bit far away and we needed to get there in order to make our flight so we went with it.

Let me tell you it was eventful. All of us laughed so much in the back on the way it was awesome. My cousin got in the car first then I did. After me was my aunt and then my mom.

There were only three seats in the back so half of my body was on my cousin and my other half was on my aunt's lap. All I can say is that it was not very comfortable for an hour-long ride.

Trying to hang on and not hurt my cousin and aunt but also get in a position where I wasn't hurting was not easy. Turns were especially hard, but we made it to the airport safely. We had a layover in Michigan and then we finally made it back to Milwaukee and drove home. From the moment we got in the car we were still laughing and having fun all the way up until the end. It was a trip that I did not expect to have as much fun and laughs as we did, and I will forever cherish this trip with the people in my life that mean a lot to me.

Every adventure and vacation in my life I have been able to grow and learn from and have shaped me into the adventurous, wild, crazy, adrenaline loving girl that I am today. I love traveling and exploring and hope to see many more places in the world. I want to continue and hopefully meet and learn new things and people along the way.

New York

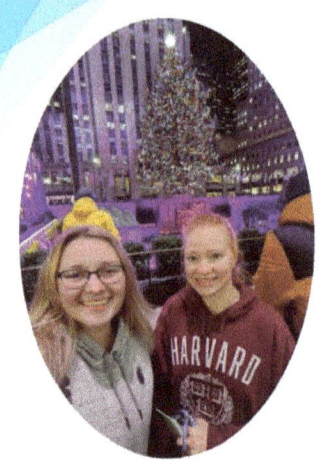

Rockefeller Plaza

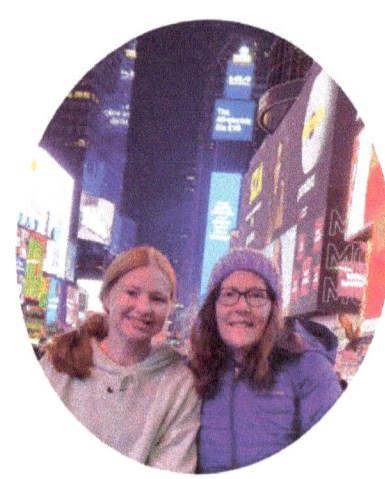

My mom and me at Times Square with the ball behind us.

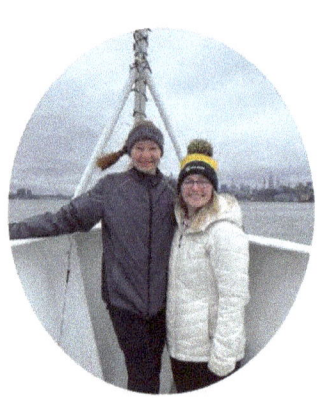

In the front of the boat on the way to see the Statue of Liberty.

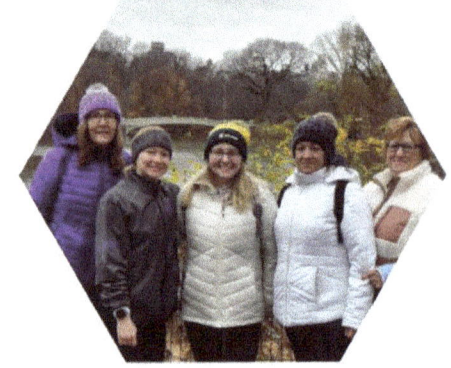

All 5 of us walking through Central Park and seeing more of NYC.

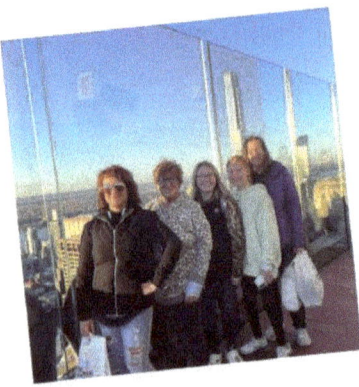

My aunt, grandma, cousin, me, and my mom at Top Of The Rock Observatory.

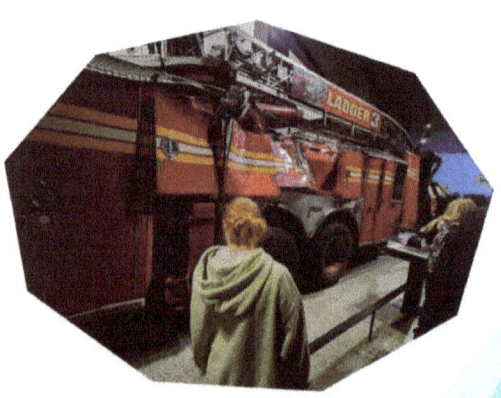

This is the very first fire truck on scene on 9/11.

Think I'M POSSIBLE

"Happiness is letting go of what you think your life is supposed to look like and celebrating it for everything that it is"

-Mandy Hale.

So many times we want things to be different and wish that we had things that other people have. Whether that be a specific hair color, house, car, eyes, etc. but when we come back to reality it just isn't that way. Are there days where I wish that I could live one day without Spina Bifida? Yes, but all the other days I live with it, and I adapt. I adapt in ways that work for me and make me a better person than I was yesterday. I've learned that in order for myself to grow I will have to be different from my friends or my family. Everyone has different aspirations for life, and everyone wants to accomplish something different in their life. In order to do that, we all need to follow the path that is best created for that. We need to find the people who are going to support that but most importantly we need to put our own work in to make those dreams happen. Our dreams and things that are most important to us in our life will not come easy. Every day everyone has *the opportunity to wake up and choose to push on or give up.* The ones who really want it will *do whatever it takes* to keep moving forward. *Set reminders, have a quote you look at every day,* do something that will allow you to go to bed at the end of the day proud of what you were able to accomplish and be ready to go again the next day. *Enjoy the journey you are on.* No one writes your story but yourself. There isn't one point in your story that says, "this is the end." There aren't any barriers that you can't get over. You will have speed bumps in your path, *but the end isn't when you are tired, it is when you are done.* If I would have stopped when I was tired, there would be thousands of "ends" in my book, including in this one but there's not. Many times, you will fail, cry, fall, embarrass yourself, get told "no", but those are the times that everyone around you will be given the real you. There was a time in High school where I was told that I couldn't walk properly by someone. Did I let that one negative comment affect me: ABSOLUTELY NOT. I moved on. If there is determination and fire inside of you, you will be able to look at those people and say, *"Bring it on, I'll prove you wrong."* I would get up and prove to those negative people who you really are and what you are capable of. Those people then are not worth your time because your true friends and family will stick with you even through your crazy ideas and adventures. They don't see and know the person you are on the inside. I like using and saying the phrase *"Suck it up."* If something is hard and tough, well *"suck it up and do it,"* if you don't want to do something because you're lazy; "suck it up" because 100% of the time I guarantee you, you will end up loving yourself for accomplishing whatever you just got done doing. Remember that *the journey you are on is a marathon not a sprint.* Everyone gets a custom medal at the end of this, you don't need to get first place to feel satisfied, you just need to be happy that you completed your goals. If you are able to eventually live your last days knowing that you gave everything in your life your all, that's what should truly matter.

"Enjoy each and every step of the journey and embrace the destination when you get there."

If there is one thing that sticks most in your mind from all of this, remember that *life may throw us all a curveball, we will be different from others, we will get knocked down, and cry multiple times but it is up to us individually on how we want our story to be written.* No one else is in control of the ship we sail but ourselves. Wake up each day and think about how you want your next page to sound like. *Live in the moment, you only live once, make it count.*

Some Messages from Friends and Family…

Being friends with Elizabeth has positively impacted my life in so many ways. After so many years, Elizabeth has shown me how important it is to get out of your comfort zone and take advantage of every opportunity. I am always so impressed by how involved Elizabeth is in powerlifting, tennis, soccer, and so much more. Also, Elizabeth is hands down the bravest person I know. She always wants to do adventurous things such as zip lining and cliff jumping. Without Elizabeth, I would never have been pushed out of my comfort zone and experienced these amazing things. I am so glad that I am friends with Elizabeth. Without her, my life would be so boring.

Kendra
(Friend)

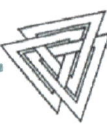
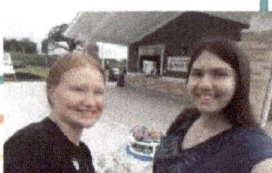

Thank you for always being at my sporting events and supporting me in everything that I have done in life. You have shown me that no matter what, I should not give up in life. Watching us grow up together, from daycare until now, has been such a special journey being so close in age. You have shown me that you should never give up and reach for the stars, no matter what you are trying to achieve. I will always be grateful for that.

Michael
(Cousin)

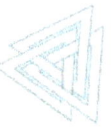
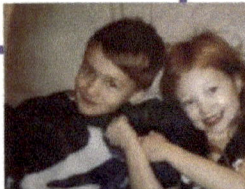

From the first moment I met Elizabeth Banes, I was in awe of her. She was a quiet, shy, petite little kindergartener with braces on both legs nestled up to her mom's legs at our first Girl Scout meeting. Upon engaging the girls in an activity and seeing how much they each could handle, I was amazed by how much each of the girls could do, but no one surprised me more than Elizabeth. She was determined to be treated just the same as everyone else. I spoke with her parents after the meeting mostly to apologize for having an activity that had so much running, and they said that I was not to change anything. That Elizabeth & her parents didn't want her to be treated any differently than anyone else. In the beginning I was very nervous about this and did try to keep physical activities at a minimum, but those were her favorite activities. As the years went by the sweet and shy girl came more and more out of her shell. She went from needing her mom for sleepovers to feeling the desperate need to go alone and embrace her own independence. As the girls all continued growing through scouts and teaching badges to each other, I became less and less surprised that Elizabeth would often pick the most physical badges that were offered for each level. She became more and more independent as well, getting into different sports such as soccer, tennis, and powerlifting. Just to name a few. On our Junior Jamboree tug of war team, she was awesome as the anchor. Her upper body strength and determination helped the whole team pull their hearts out! I must admit that she was an inspiration to me personally as well. I was diagnosed with MS in 2008 and often hid that information from new friends and acquaintances- because I didn't want to be treated differently. I didn't ever want someone to exclude me from being asked to lend a helping hand because of my condition. I also never wanted to regret someday when my health really deteriorated that I didn't do all I could for my own two daughters and the over two dozen Girl Scout daughters I have had over the years to better their lives and help them grow into the amazing woman they are destined to become. Where I am able to "hide" my disability, Elizabeth is not. She has had to overcome obstacles that most people cannot even comprehend. I think that might be why we both enjoy teasing each other so much. Over the years, I know as a troop leader, we shouldn't have favorites, but she is definitely one of my top 10!

Jen
(Troop Leader)

The day you were born, we both (while working) sat by our phones to hear that you had arrived. That day was so special. Your dad told us that you came out screaming and kicking your legs and that you had red hair. We knew right then you would be special and that you were a fighter. We loved watching you swim and tried to help you, but your parents said, "She needs to learn to do it on her own" (which I felt so bad for you). But looking back now, I can totally see their point, and they were right. I feel that if you didn't learn to do things on your own you wouldn't have done anything at all. You and I always had a special bond (no matter what it was) until Uncle Jesse came into the picture, and then it was you and Uncle Jesse. He always told me, and still does say, that you and him have the best bond. The summers that you spent at our house and us riding our bikes around town to get exercise were awesome. Those days were the best! I can't believe that you are a senior in high school and how fast these years have gone. We look forward to seeing you reach for the stars and become awesome. We love you so much, and when God made you he definitely broke the mold. Also, remember, day or night we are always here for you with anything that you need.

Alicia & Jesse
(Aunt & Uncle)

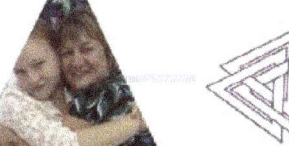

I've known Elizabeth since we were babies in daycare. She was probably my first-ever friend. My favorite thing about Elizabeth is that she never lets anything stop her from doing what she really wants to do. She lifts heavy weights (that gives her muscles I'm pretty jealous of), plays soccer, and is super active. You wouldn't even think she has a disability. I also love her "You only live once mindset." She's not afraid to take a few risks and jump off a cliff two or three times. When I think about Elizabeth, my first thought is never about her disability, but instead, it's being thankful that I have a lifelong friend who inspires me every day.

Abbey
(Friend)

You have always supported me; in school, coming to my events, moving out of state. know even though we have our brother/sister moments where we argue or don't get along that we have a true commitment to one another. We care about each other an will always support one another. You are honest with me and push me to do more and be my best. I love that you never let your birth defect stop you. You meet challenge head-on and say no, I'm not doing that. I'm doing it my way. If I didn't have you in my life, I wouldn't be traumatized from ocean vacations where you made me go on a banana boat, dolphin & whale watching, or parasailing to have a seal jump out of the water at me. However, without you there are many experiences I wouldn't have had. am very proud to be your brother. I will be with you every step of the way, whereve your future takes you. I know you will do great things, Elizabeth. Love you.

Noah
(Brother)

Elizabeth, when you asked me to write about the impact you have had on my life, and I started thinking about it, I decided it's more about how you have not impacted my life. My life wouldn't be the same without you. I see your beautiful face in the morning and hear you say I love you, and I am thankful you are mine. My life is full of love, adventure, kindness, humor and absolute pure joy because of you. You inspire me every day and make me appreciate the little things in life. My concern right from day one was that you were the best you and that you were happy and healthy... that was all that mattered and still is. Any expectation that anyone has had for you, you have surpassed. Right from the very beginning, with rolling over, crawling, pulling yourself up, walking... the infamous story of you zipping around the living room with the walker and then pushing it away. That is the heart of who you are...that determination that I can do it if I set my mind to it. That inspires me. You inspire me to try new things and to keep going when things are difficult. You do you so well that people forget you even have a birth defect. I know nothing is easy for you and no one but you will truly know what you go through or experience day to day but you don't let that stop you. You have an inner strength, and let that push you even more. Your belief in yourself is one of your greatest strengths. Right from the beginning we decided we were not going to treat you any different than brother. You should be expected to at least try something, then if you couldn't do it, ok but you were not starting with that attitude. Man, did you live up to that? Always know you have my complete love and support. You make me so proud every day to say that you are my daughter. It isn't even about everything you accomplish; it's about who you are as a person. You are the kindest, most loving soul that I know. Having you in my life inspires me to be a better mom and person, to try harder, be more accepting and kinder to others. I always think, 'As my daughter says, you only live once. How you push yourself to be the best in whatever you do inspires me. You give 110% to whatever you do. Working at the camp, you are the hardest worker and always do things for everyone. Exercising, you are always trying new things-, running and always pushing yourself harder or to do more, to do better. School, you are willing to try different classes or activities, to meet new people, and never letting it stop you that you don't know anyone participating: tennis, powerlifting, soccer, NHS. Girl Scouts, all the trips and things you have gotten to do (cliff jumping, Chicago, Mall of America). Even the Junior Jamboree competitions where you were the anchor for the tug of war! Now, writing your book and going for your gold award. Coming to terms with your disability and going to all the doctor appointments, talking with the doctors, and doing all the tests. I love that you talk with people about it and are so open because it means that you are accepting of it and of yourself. Writing this book was a big step- for the amount of work it is, the amount of time it's taken, and for revealing your innermost thoughts & feelings to the world. I cannot wait to see the finished product and you can be so proud of yourself. We call you our 'adventure coordinator,' and that title is true for life, not just vacations. Before you, we knew nothing about Spina Bifida. We had no idea what we would have to do, how to go about it, how we would help you, or what life had in store for you. We have taken every step together, the four of us, with you leading us. From daycare to starting school, then moving to middle school & high school- we never knew what was coming. Now, the current adventure of college tours/deciding on a college and moving you off on your own to discover your own life. The vacations that none of us will forget, where you inspire all of us to go way beyond our comfort zones: roller coasters, gator tours, jet boats on the ocean, banana boats, parasailing, kayaking at night, jet skis. We all 'suck it up' because we don't want to disappoint you. If Elizabeth wants to do it, then I am going to try it for her, inspired by her bravery and zest for life. I love you beyond words and just seeing your beautiful face every day makes me smile. I am thankful every day that God gave me you, and I can be part of your journey. You always make me laugh, and I love watching you navigate through life- be it your sports, studies, your life decisions... to see how you are growing and maturing and the adult decisions you are making. The sky is the limit, my girl, and I cannot wait to see where your journey leads. You are my greatest blessing and my best friend. Love, Mom.

Kristen
(Mom)

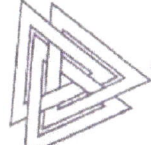

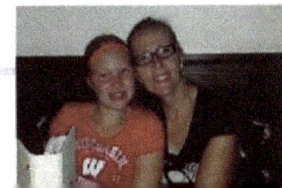

Since day 1, like Noah, the first time I saw you, that red hair, I knew I was in for the trip of a lifetime. thought, "Oh boy!" Since that day, you have done nothing but inspire me in everything I do. Even the famo quotes you have brought to our family, "Suck it Up!" "Use your resources wisely!" and most important, "Yo only live once!" The smile you started your life with impacted everyone around you, including me. A girl, w didn't know how life would be for you, and you just kept pushing the envelope. From rolling over to crawlir to pulling yourself up, pushing away your walker at 3 (I got this!). Showing that smile and making me smile with joy. Growing up, you have always had the purest heart and have never thought you needed any specic help. That made your mom and I so proud. You were independent, and that showed me that it is how you approached every day. That is truly inspirational to me. All that and then there are all the new things yo have brought into our lives, the different adventures. Only you would bring that to me and this family. Th famous phrase "I want to do that." You have shown, and keep showing me, how to have fun and take every chance you can, try something new and have that adventure. "You only live once!" From parasailing, banan boat rides, jet skis (oh boy, the jet ski!. Yelling at me to go faster), and all the adventures. You have inspired me in so many ways. Have fun when you can, and smile every day while having that fun. Every day you make me think of the adventures I will have today and smile at them no matter what. As you get olde and embark on your next day, you have made me look to you for my next inspiration. I know you will have o With all that you have done and said and not said, I feel you think it all the time, and that is the biggest inspiration you have had on me, and I will hold it for the rest of my life. "Tell me it will be hard to do or th I can't do it! I will prove you wrong, I will do it," and with those inspirations you have made in the short ti so far, you have impacted my life from the worries to the proud moments you have yourself and yourself alone. Thank you forever and ever and all the people you have impacted and inspired!

Derrick
(Dad)

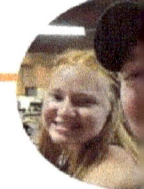

I've watched you over the years not let anything stand in your way, and whatever you want, you go out and get it. You don't take NO for an answer. I can't wait to see what else you do in this world.

Lauren
(Cousin)

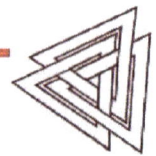

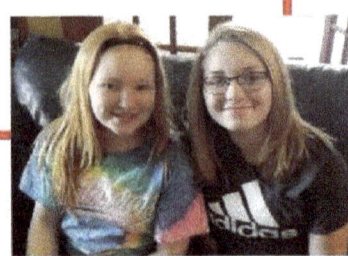

You are such a joy to all of us. We remember when we found out that you would have a disability that we knew very little about. It was scary, really scary, but with prayer and the decision your parents made, we would all do whatever it took to have you part of our family, make sure you were happy, and make many memories. The day you were born, holding you for the first time, was so beautiful. That red hair really sets the pace for your personality. Your spunkiness, determination, your facial expressions just kept us all going. The first time you walked away from your walker just made us all cry. Your mom picked you up from daycare, and you walked to her away from your walker. She called all of us to tell us the most wonderful news. We were told the best thing we could do for you was let you do everything yourself. You got a little spunky but we all tried to be firm, but it was hard for grandma and grandpa to see you struggle at times, but that helped you become more independent. There were times you would fall and jump right back up and say, "I'm ok, I got it," and never cried. Your many Drs. were always amazed at your progress. Then school started. You wanted to try everything and whatever it took, and you did it. We were so proud of you for all your sports, academics, and all your achievements. With the help of your mom and dad, you were encouraged to try whatever your heart desired. You never disappointed us. It was so much fun going to all your daycare concerts and programs, and we could pick you out of the group- yes, the red hair. So beautiful. Everyone knew you were Elizabeth. Then Girl Scouts- we are so pleased you worked so hard those many years, selling Girl Scouts cookies, going on field trips, horseback riding, jumping off of cliffs to the water below with no fear. There was nothing you wouldn't try. Bowling, tennis, soccer, powerlifting, and on and on. We tried to make every meet, every game, every social event that we could and sitting in the stands feeling so very proud of you. So many times, we would go by your house and you were out running, jogging to help build strength. Even the campers at the campground would be in awe when you were out running laps around the park to build your strength. Eating healthy & exercising & determination not to give up was a big part of your growth. Oh, then you got inducted into the National Honors Society. Wow, we all said, "No one in our family was ever in the National Honors Society." We all were so proud. All your volunteering and hard work, your determination, and just being you made you shine even more. Now, you will be going off to college in a year. The sky is the limit, and you will reach it, no doubt. Never let anyone tell you you can't do something because we know you will prove them wrong over and over again. Love you, E!

Adrian & Charlene
(Grandpa & Grandma)

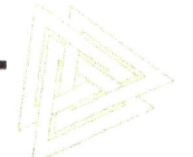
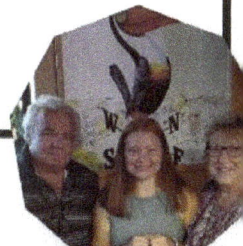

Additional Facts

People with Spina Bifida have a harder time organizing things and lose things more often.

Children with Spina Bifida have a hard time paying attention in class or in general.

Kids with Spina Bifida struggle to be able to read, write, move and use tools due to lack of hand-eye coordination.

Most kids diagnosed with Spina Bifida struggle with math and math procedures.

It can be difficult for people with Spina Bifida to plan things out and have a set schedule.

Half of the people living with Spina Bifida in the US are adults.

166,000 individuals in the US are diagnosed with Spina Bifida.

Spina Bifida occurs in 1 of every 2,758 births.

80% of people with Spina Bifida have Hydrocephalus- an excessive amount of spinal fluid on the brain and a shunt is required to be put in.

Everyday there are about 8 babies in the US who are born with Spina Bifida or something similar.

Spina Bifida is the most commonly permantely disabiling birth defect in life.

The average length that a baby diagnosed with Spina Bifida stays in the NICU is 2 weeks.

www.ingramcontent.com/pod-product-compliance
Lightning Source LLC
Chambersburg PA
CBHW051207120626
46547CB00013B/1244